Growing up with Parents who have Learning Difficulties

Tim Booth and Wendy Booth

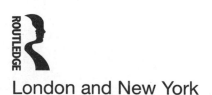

London and New York

First published 1998
by Routledge
11 New Fetter Lane, London EC4P 4EE

Simultaneously published in the USA and Canada
by Routledge
29 West 35th Street, New York, NY 10001

Typeset in Baskerville by Routledge
Printed and bound in Great Britain by MPG Books Ltd, Bodmin

British Library Cataloguing in Publication Data
A catalogue record for this book is available from the British Library

Library of Congress Cataloguing in Publication Data
Growing up with parents who have learning difficulties/Tim Booth and
Wendy Booth.
Includes bibliographical references and index.
1. Parenting 2. Learning disabilities. 3. Children of handicapped parents. I.
Booth, Wendy. II. Title.
HQ755.8.B657   1998
306.874–dc21   97-41065
                                                                    CIP

ISBN 0–415–16655–1 (hbk)
ISBN 0–415–16656–x (pbk)

To the memory of Ann Craft who showed so many the way

Contents

Acknowledgements

First came the idea. At that point we were unsure whether the study we had in mind would prove feasible. We didn't know if it would be possible to trace the now-adult children of parents with learning difficulties, how to go about doing so, or whether they would consent to take part. The University of Sheffield agreed to fund Wendy Booth for three months to find out. Without this support, we might never have taken the idea forward and we certainly wouldn't have been able to draft such a well-grounded research proposal.

We are indebted to the Joseph Rowntree Foundation for funding the study and for giving us the freedom and opportunity to pursue our interest in narrative research in the learning difficulties field.

The task of tracking down our subjects took us into a range of voluntary and statutory agencies in Sheffield, Kirklees, Derbyshire, Barnsley, Oldham, Bradford, Wakefield, Rotherham, Leeds, Calderdale, Rochdale and Nottingham. It is impossible to name individually all the people in all these places who in some way put themselves about for us, but without their help it is unlikely the study would ever have got done.

We are also grateful to Steve Dowson, Danny Goodley, Richard Jenkins, Sharon Macdonald and Michael Rodgers for reading and commenting on some of the draft chapters, and to Jill Kerkhoff whose accurate and skilful transcribing of the taped interviews made our work so much easier.

The Family Policy Studies Centre and the editor of *Disability and Society* kindly gave their permission for us to draw on material originally published in an earlier draft by them.

Our sons, Matthew and Daniel, helped to keep our work in perspective and to remind us in their own inimitable ways that parenting does not end when the children grow up.

Lastly, our thanks go to all the people who opened their doors to us and opened their hearts too. Most of all, we hope you approve of what we have done with your stories.

Chapter 1

Introduction

This book is about the stories of people who grew up in families where at least one parent had learning difficulties.

At one level, it is a book about parenting by mothers and fathers with learning difficulties as seen through the eyes, and judged by what has become, of their now-adult children. It is also about growing up with a disabled parent or parents, and, hopefully, it goes some way to meeting what Buck and Hohmann (1983) identified as a 'dire need for further research' into children's adjustment to parental disability. But the relevance of the study extends beyond the immediate group of parents to which it refers. Surprisingly little is known about what constitutes good-enough parenting or about the relationship between parental competence, family functioning and child outcomes. Looking at out-of-the-ordinary families throws new light on taken-for-granted assumptions about the process of parenting. Parents who break the rules help to define them more clearly. Observing children under pressure shows up the extent of their adaptability. Studying parenting on the margins of competence provides a new perspective on the limits of parental adequacy.

There are no reliable estimates of the number of parents with learning difficulties. Their true prevalence is unknown and probably unknowable. They represent a still largely invisible population. There is no list or register. Conducting any sort of count is well nigh impossible in practical terms. At the margin, they merge into the general population. Most sources agree, however, that the number of people with learning difficulties who become parents is steadily growing, and will continue to do so, as a result of hospital closures, decreased segregation, changing attitudes towards sexuality and wider opportunities for independent living and participation in the community. Parenthood may be seen as both a choice and a consequence of ordinary living. As and when people with learning difficulties are freed from invasive control of their own sexuality so more of them will have children. The same trend has been reported in Britain, America, Australia, Canada, Denmark and Germany. The need for a better understanding of the consequences for children of growing up in such families and of how their parents might best be supported becomes ever more urgent as their numbers rise.

Parents with learning difficulties are widely presumed to present a high risk of parenting breakdown. Successive studies have reported high rates (40–60 per cent) for the removal of children from the family home (Accardo and Whitman, 1990; Cross and Marks, 1995; New York State Commission on Quality of Care for the Mentally Disabled, 1993b; Scally, 1973). Research also suggests that the children of parents with learning difficulties are at risk of developmental delay, maltreatment, neglect and abuse (Schilling et al., 1982). This evidence has contributed to the view that people with learning difficulties lack the competence to provide good-enough parenting. Oliver (1977), for example, asserts that they 'continue to be incompetent rearers, whatever supportive treatment is offered', and Fotheringham (1980) too claims that few parents have the ability to provide 'conditions of care at the minimal acceptable level'. Accardo and Whitman (1990) argue that the only important question 'with regard to parenting failure of significantly mentally retarded adults would seem to be not whether but when'.

The study on which this book is based arose directly from earlier work in which we documented the lives and struggles of parents with learning difficulties through personal accounts of their own experience of child-rearing and parenthood (Booth and Booth, 1994a). This research showed that such blanket judgements of parental incompetence are not grounded in the lives of parents themselves. The statistics on child removal owe as much to the decisions of professionals and the courts as to the behaviour of parents. The fact is that people with learning difficulties frequently fall victim to an expectation of parental inadequacy that is made real through the decisions and actions of those with the power to intervene in their lives. This 'presumption of incompetence' renders parents with learning difficulties vulnerable to discriminatory treatment and prejudicial judgements about their ability to cope with the demands of parenthood. From this point of view, parental competence is not just an attribute of the person but an attributed status that reflects the normative standards used for defining good-enough parenting by those charged with making the assessments

(Booth and Booth, 1996a, 1996b). Another crucial factor working against parents with learning difficulties is the emphasis currently given to the protection of children at the expense of their broader welfare needs and the support of their families (Farmer and Owen, 1993; Parton, 1991; Thorpe, 1995).

A common response to this research was that we had argued a case for parents that did not take account of the interests or welfare of their children (Schofield, 1996). What, people wanted to know, becomes of children who grow up in such families? This study began as an attempt to address this question.

Almost nothing is known about the grown-up children of parents with learning difficulties. There has been no longitudinal research on the effects of being raised by a parent or parents who have learning difficulties (Tymchuk and Feldman, 1991), and no attempt has yet been made to chart their children's progress through adolescence and into adulthood (Dowdney and Skuse, 1993; New York State Commission on Quality of Care for the Mentally Disabled, 1993b). Consequently, 'little can be said as yet about the long-term effects of parenting' by people with learning difficulties (Zetlin *et al.*, 1985). The problems of tracking them down and eliciting their co-operation have stalled investigation and deterred researchers who, instead, have focused their attention on more get-at-able infants and toddlers. Most studies have been attached to early intervention programmes that focus mainly on families with young children aged from birth to three years (Tymchuk, 1990a). This fact has not stopped people from speculating about the longer-term risks of such an upbringing. They have simply projected the developmental deficits observed and assessed among young children into later life. The result makes for some gloomy prognostications. Accardo and Whitman (1990), for example, suggest that parents' difficulties 'in meeting the developmental and behavioral needs of pre-school children seem to intensify and become insurmountable with late school-age children and adolescents.' Consequently, the children are presumed to grow into less than competent adults for want of the example and guidance they need in order to mature properly (McFadyean, 1995).

Such ideas illustrate what Wolin and Wolin (1995) have called 'damage model thinking'. The damage model portrays children from troubled homes as helpless victims whose struggle against the odds eventually takes its toll in forms of pathological adaptation in adolescence and adulthood. Several considerations counsel against making any simple connections between the quality of parenting received in childhood and the quality of life enjoyed in adulthood. For a start, mothers and fathers are not the only people who are involved in bringing up children (Rapoport *et al.*, 1977). Other parent-figures – family, friends, neighbours, professional helpers – can provide cover where mum and dad are stretched, and the family support system can compensate for shortcomings in the skills of parents to ensure adequate care for the child (Tymchuk, 1992). Also, it has long been known that some children exhibit a resilience in the face of adversity and manage to thrive despite poor care and lives filled with difficulty. In any case, parenting is not a one-way street. Children themselves play an active part in seeking out and constructing environments that sustain their needs (Werner, 1993). People's destinies are not laid down in early childhood. Early learning certainly exerts a crucial influence on development but it may also be modified as a result of later experience (Rutter, 1974). Lastly, 'damage model thinking' easily gives way to a self-fulfilling prophecy on the part of professionals who, pessimistic about the prospects for the child, fail to support the parents and so bring about the outcomes they fear. All these factors suggest that the relationship between parental competence and child outcomes across the life cycle is far more complicated than the damage model allows. A key aim of this study was to try to unravel this knot through the lives of now-adult children brought up in families widely judged to operate on the edge of competence.

The research was designed to explore four main themes:

- What does it mean to be brought up by a parent or parents with learning difficulties?
- Does being raised by parents with learning difficulties affect children's well-being and adjustment in later life?
- How do children cope with their parents' learning difficulties?
- Is there a clear link between parental competence and child outcomes?

We have chosen to use narrative methods for tackling our task, by which we mean methods aimed at depicting people's subjective experience in ways that are faithful to the meaning they give to their lives. Narrative methods vary in their forms and purposes. The purest form of narrative is the *autobiography* where the subject is also the sole author. *Reminiscence* is the unstructured recalling of past events and feelings without any attempt to be inclusive or thorough about the life course. *Life review* is a process of reflection in which people appraise their own past from their standpoint in the present. The *life story* is a collaborative account of all or part of an individual's life, delivered orally by that person to an amanuensis. The *life history* subsumes the life story but also includes biographical information from a range of other sources.

These narrative forms may serve a variety of uses. For example, adapting Abrams (1991) slightly, five overlapping categories of narrative may be identified. *First-person agony narratives* recount painful experiences as a means of challenging the moral or social order through the sympathies or conscience of the reader (see, for example, Ashe (1989) who weaves her own experience of childbirth into an examination of the legal regulation of reproduction). *Insider narratives* aim to provide an insight into subjective worlds beyond the reader's ken (see, for example, Lewis' (1961) classic account of family life in a Mexican slum). *Grounded narratives* render abstract ideas accessible in terms of everyday human experience (see, for example, Williams (1991) on racism). *Fringe narratives* give voice to previously unheard or suppressed perspectives (see, for example, Jane Fry's account of her life as a transsexual in Bogdan (1974), or Parker (1991) on 'lifers'). Finally, *mould-breaking narratives* help to reformulate a problem, cast something in a new light or otherwise change our understanding (see, for example, Warshaw (1989) on the date rape phenomenon).

Despite this variety, narrative methods display a number of common characteristics:

- They provide an 'inner view of the person' (Birren and Deutchman, 1991) by treating people as 'expert witnesses' in the matter of their own lives whose stories can provide a point of entry into their world through the imagination of the reader.
- They are a means of making abstract claims more tangible by grounding them in concrete lived experience.
- They help to counteract the problem of the 'disappearing individual' in sociological theorising where the search for abstraction and generalisation often renders people into little more than ciphers, and leads both scholars and students to lose sight of human individuals as a creative force in the making of their own lives and their own history.
- They form a bridge between the individual and society by giving access through people's lives to structural features of their social world. By 'listening beyond' (Bertaux-Wiame, 1981) the words of any particular informant, it is possible to pick up the echoes of other people's experience and to identify the themes that make them also the stories of a group. These common threads connecting people's accounts reveal how their lives are shaped by the wider society and throw light on the network of social relations to which they belong.

In this way, as Ferrarotti (1981) has observed, the 'effort to understand a biography in all its uniqueness . . . becomes the effort to interpret a social system'.

Three considerations have influenced our decision to adopt a narrative approach. First, there is no sampling frame for the focus group of adult children, and no possibility of guaranteeing the representativeness required for statistical generalisation. Indeed, the task of identifying, locating and securing the co-operation of subjects within this largely hidden population presents major logistical hurdles that have thwarted or deterred retrospective research in this field. Second, more structured methods of research run the risk of oversimplifying people's stories and imposing order and meaning on lives that are 'more ambiguous, more problematic, and more chaotic in reality' (Faraday and Plummer, 1979). Third, the methodological problems of trying to establish a causal connection between family processes and later outcomes for people brought up by parents with learning difficulties are probably insurmountable. The use of narrative methods opens up the possibility of establishing a bridge using people's subjective interpretation of their own lived experience. We have tried throughout the book to pay attention to the research issues raised by our study, and especially to what Lincoln and Denzin (1994) have called the problems of 'representation' and 'legitimation' presented by the narrative approach. We have also tried to experiment with ways of reporting our material that confront the challenge of doing narrative research with inarticulate subjects (Booth, 1995). Indeed, in writing a book about the stories told us by now-adult children of parents with learning difficulties, we like to think that we have also produced a text about the making of a narrative.

The chapters that follow are largely free-standing and, with the exception of chapter 7, which offers an analysis and commentary on the material presented in chapter 6, may be read in any order without detriment to the sense of the whole. Each provides a different angle on the same theme. Taken together, we have tried to present a sympathetic portrayal of what it means to grow up with a parent who has learning difficulties; one that is true to the experience it seeks to convey. Chapter 2 describes how the research was conducted and the difficulties it presented, and provides an overview of the people and families involved in the study. Given that half the informants in the study themselves had learning difficulties, chapter 3 addresses the challenge of undertaking narrative research with inarticulate subjects. Chapter 4 looks at how the people in the study managed the transition to adulthood, drawing on empirical indicators and evidence about the quality of their lives. Chapter 5 examines why some children overcome the adversities of their childhood and upbringing where others succumb, and considers how competence may be sustained by a supportive environment. Chapter 6 presents a personal narrative about growing up with a mother who has learning difficulties in the form of a first-person dialogue between two sisters. Chapter 7 provides an analysis and interpretation of the wider significance of the sisters' story. Chapter 8 offers a critical appraisal of the notion of 'reverse dependency' or 'role reversal' as a supposed feature of relationships between disabled parents and their children. Chapter 9 shows the disabling effects that system abuse can have on families and illustrates the role that advocacy can play in enabling them to resist its threat. Chapter 10 draws out some of the implications of the study for policy and practice in supporting families in their parenting.

Chapter 2

Doing the research

In this chapter we describe how the research was done, the problems we encountered on the way, and the characteristics of our study group.

The target group identified for inclusion in the study comprised men and women aged (preferably) between eighteen and thirty years who had spent the greater part of their childhood living in a family where one or both parents had learning difficulties.

For research purposes, parents were held to satisfy the inclusion criteria if they were known to have received health, education or social services specifically designated for use by people with learning difficulties at some time in their lives, or if a professional who knew them personally confirmed that they had been so labelled. This was the only practical approach in the circumstances given that the parents themselves were not the subjects of the research, many were not seen or contacted and some were now dead. The expedient of using a person's current or former status as a service user as a surrogate for unobtainable test or clinical data in order to establish their learning difficulties has both a theoretical rationale (Mercer, 1973) and an administrative precedent, being the method used by many health authorities to identify those who are eligible for registration with their case registers (Farmer *et al.*, 1993).

The decision to target adult children in the eighteen to thirty age range was taken because we wanted respondents who were able to look back and reflect on their own childhood and upbringing from a position in the adult world, but whose memories were not too far distant from the events and experiences they described. Things did not quite turn out as planned. Difficulties in locating willing subjects and the way the introductions and interviews were set up (see below) meant that a number of younger and older people were admitted to the study. All in all, eighteen of the thirty subjects fell within the prescribed band while two were below-age and ten were over-age.

The research questions driving the study required that the adult children who took part had grown up mostly in the care of their parents at home, and had maintained contact with their family during any spell away from home. This requirement seriously limited the pool of eligible subjects. Research has pointed to high rates (40–60 per cent) for the removal of children from the family home. Of the twenty families involved in our earlier study of parents with learning difficulties (Booth and Booth, 1994a), fourteen had had one or more of their children placed in short-term or permanent care. Twenty to thirty years ago, when our prospective subjects were born, it is arguably even less likely than today that the interests of the child would have been seen as best served by remaining in a family headed by parent(s) with learning difficulties.

Many adult children were located who had spent too long away from their parents to qualify for inclusion in the study. In the context of people's family lives it is not surprising that grown-up children with relatively secure and stable home backgrounds were hard to find. Crises of family survival precipitated by poverty, broken relationships or official intervention were pandemic. Only half (fifteen) of the study group had remained at home in the care of at least one parent with learning difficulties until they came of age or until they moved out to live independently. Five of our subjects had spent less than two years away from their parent(s), and a further three had been in care for two to four years. Of the remaining seven, all had spent more than four years in children's homes or residential schools but had remained in contact with their parents throughout this period. The majority of this group (five) had spent at least ten years of their childhood with their parent(s). The shortest time that anyone had lived at home was seven years, although in this case the lad went home from his residential school for weekends and holidays.

LOCATING THE SUBJECTS

Adult children of parents with learning difficulties constitute a hidden population for research purposes. There is no register of names through which they can be traced. Tracking them down presents the same problems as trying to trace the children of, say, parents who cannot read or write, or children whose mothers are tone deaf. There are too few to identify them through a general trawl of the population, and in any case such an approach would not be feasible given the sensitive nature of the subject and the difficulties of verifying people's responses. Consideration was given to placing a feature about the study in the local press inviting people to come forward but this idea was rejected because again there would be no way of validating the parents' status, and also for reasons of interviewer safety.

The only practical means of overcoming these enumeration problems was to trace possible subjects through parents known to the services. Even this method was far from straightforward. Some professionals were noticeably reluctant or unwilling to label people as having learning difficulties. Data protection restrictions limit the possibilities for searching the records held by service agencies and in any case information about people's adult children was rarely available on file. No agency was in a position to supply a list of people with learning difficulties known to have children aged between eighteen to thirty years. Legal hurdles aside, such information was usually known only to individual practitioners about individual clients. Accordingly, people working in the learning difficulties services were approached personally and asked if they knew directly or indirectly of any parents with adult children, or knew of anyone else who might know such a parent.

This method of using such 'key informants' (Whitman and Accardo, 1990) has a number of weaknesses. It excludes people who are not known to the service agencies; possibly over-represents the less competent parents or those with greater problems and fewer community supports; and is very time-consuming. Any bias resulting from the first two problems is likely to be small. Most parents with learning difficulties will probably come to the attention of the statutory services at some time when their children are growing up. The other limitation must be seen as part of the price for doing the research at all.

The key informant method took us into twelve local authority areas in search of our target quota of adult children. Enquiries were pursued and leads followed up through social workers and social services teams, adult training centres and social education centres, special schools, special needs tutors in further education colleges, community nurses and community learning disability teams, local case registers, clinical psychologists, educational psychologists, careers officers, Family Service Units, a range of voluntary organisations and other personal contacts. The task of locating our subjects turned out to be a major logistical venture, and the difficulties we encountered were one of the main reasons why the fieldwork stage of the research took fifteen months to complete instead of the eight months we had initially planned. The process was more like private detective work than research sampling: more Raymond Chandler than Moser and Kalton. It involved tracking down sources, cold calling, getting a foot in the door, following up leads, checking out information, blundering down blind alleys, cultivating informants, using go-betweens and a great deal of legwork in pursuit of what in research terms were the equivalent of missing persons. Even so, obtaining the names of potential subjects was only the first step to establishing contact.

ESTABLISHING CONTACT

Finding the names of parents with learning difficulties known to have grown-up children was only a port of call on route to our final destination. The next stage was to find out where the children lived and to arrange for an introduction. This was not so easy as it sounds. The sources who had come up with the parent(s)' names were not always acquainted with the children, did not always know their home address and anyway could not usually divulge such information for reasons of confidentiality. In any case, given the nature of the study and the vulnerabilities of the families, we felt it was important that the initial approach should be made via people who were familiar and accountable, and in a way that left the initiative with the subject.

A number of leads fizzled out at this stage or had to be dropped. Some parents were found to have died and their children's whereabouts were unknown, or the children had left home and lost contact with their parents. Other grown-up children had emigrated or now lived in another part of the country. In a few cases the workers involved advised that family circumstances militated against the research (for example, because of a recent bereavement, illness, mental health problems or a pending court case) or that the individual concerned was unable to communicate well enough to be interviewed. Some professionals refused to act as an intermediary or were instructed not to help us by their line managers. It is not possible to be sure how many potential subjects were lost in these ways, because the number of adult children in the family obviously could not be verified in every case, but at least fifteen families headed by a parent or parents with learning difficulties and known to have adult children slipped through the net before any attempt to contact them could be made.

Putting aside these setbacks, our principal line of approach was to establish contact through the good offices of an intermediary or third party already known to the person. In most cases this was a professional worker, although parents themselves or siblings were also used in this role. The only occasions when a third party was not used were where the subject was already linked into the researchers' network. Some examples will help to illustrate how the process worked in practice in particular cases:

Marie Summers

A young man with learning difficulties who satisfied the criteria for admission to the study was identified through a local case register. A member of the register's staff visited the private family placement where he lived but he was out. His carer felt he would not be co-operative but, she said, she also had a young woman living with her, Marie, whose mother had learning difficulties, whom she felt sure would be willing to take part. She offered to ask Marie. When the researcher phoned later, the carer reported that Marie was indeed quite happy to be interviewed but would prefer to meet at the FE college she attended. The carer passed on the name and telephone number of Marie's tutor at college. The researcher phoned the tutor, explained the research and asked if it would be possible to set up a quiet room for a talk. The tutor rang back to confirm the arrangements and, on the day fixed for the first interview, Marie met the researcher in the college's reception.

Peter Fenton

Peter was one of several people identified through a local case register. The register staff first wrote to his social worker outlining the study and requesting that she ask if Peter would be interested in taking part. When Peter agreed, the social worker passed on his home address and the name of the drop-in centre where he could be found most days. After several unsuccessful phone calls to the centre, the researcher stopped by at Peter's flat, only to find him out. She then wrote naming a day and time when she'd call again and asking him to let her know if it wasn't convenient. He was at home when she arrived – although he'd not received the letter.

Tina Wimpenny

Contact was made with a Community Learning Disability Team and the researcher was invited to talk about the project at a team meeting. One of the practitioners present said she knew a woman who attended

a local Adult Training Centre whose mother also had learning difficulties. The ATC manager was approached and briefed about the study.
He agreed to ask her if she'd be willing to take part. When phoned a
few days later he confirmed that she'd said yes, and wished to be seen at
the Centre.

Sandra West

A contact in Nottingham put the researcher in touch with a psychologist in Derby who arranged an introduction to a community nurse who
knew a mother with learning difficulties. The community nurse was well
acquainted with the family and asked one of the daughters, Maggie, if
she'd be willing to see the researcher. Maggie agreed and the community nurse passed on her telephone number. When she was contacted to
fix an appointment, Maggie happened to mention her sister, Sandra,
and the researcher asked if she might like to come along too. Maggie
said she'd ask and when the researcher arrived for the first interview
they were both there waiting.

Adam Lloyd

The Community Learning Disabilities Team was aware that a woman
who attended a local Adult Training Centre had a son but no-one knew
where he lived. The researcher rang the ATC manager to explain what
the research was about and to elicit his help. Without further ado he
fetched the mother herself to the phone. She was keen for her son to be
involved and, without being asked, gave his address. The researcher
wrote saying that she expected he'd heard from his mother that
someone would be contacting him, and that she'd be in the area on
Monday and would call in if it was convenient. When she arrived,
Adam and his partner were expecting her.

Where the third party was a professional or practitioner they were
usually sent a brief outline of the study explaining what it was about
and what it would involve, together with some notes aimed at antici-
pating any questions the subject might ask. They were left to decide
when, where and how best to broach the matter. Initially people were
simply asked if they would agree to see the researcher to talk about the
project. They were told that participation was entirely voluntary and
they could pull out at any time. Once consent was obtained the intermediary would either fix up a meeting at a time and place of the

subject's choosing or seek permission to pass on the person's name and address to the researcher for arrangements to be made direct. In many cases (twelve), the third party came along to make the introductions at the first meeting.

The use of intermediaries in this way has its disadvantages. The researcher has no direct control over how the study is first presented and explained; people's feelings towards the third party might act as an uncontrollable source of response bias; and, where a practitioner is involved as the go-between, the researcher may be too closely identified with authority or officialdom. In practice, there was no way round these dangers if the study was going to get done.

Our previous research led us to anticipate that some parents might feel threatened by our enquiries. Most were likely to have experienced long-term surveillance from the statutory services, persistent intervention in their private lives, and various forms of system abuse (Booth and Booth, 1995). These experiences can foster an understandable insecurity and defensiveness. We offered to meet any parents who were made anxious or suspicious by our work, or who just wanted to know more about what we were doing. Third party intermediaries were made aware of our readiness to follow up such concerns. In effect, we allowed the parents a veto over the research: we would not proceed with the interviews if they were opposed even though their son or daughter had agreed to see us. In the event, sixteen parents from eleven families were briefed personally about the study of whom two exercised their right of veto, in both cases after the first interview.

The process of establishing contact maintained a distance between researcher and subject until the latter's consent had been obtained. The third parties who acted as go-betweens had no cause to put any pressure on the people they approached and no obvious interest in trying hard to recruit them for the study. Equally the people themselves had no obvious incentive to take part in the study. On the contrary, there are many reasons why they might have preferred not to talk about a childhood that was likely to have been troubled. Both of these considerations pointed to the likelihood of a high refusal rate even when a possible subject had been tracked down. In fact, at least twelve people declined an invitation to participate in the study – around one in three of those approached.

Financial incentives in the form of a cash payment were offered in a few cases where a refusal came after an initial introduction had been made. The decision to offer a fee for interview was prompted by the difficulties of locating subjects and the costs to the project in terms of time spent in searching for a replacement. Payment was only mooted where people appeared unsure about whether or not to commit themselves. For example, in two cases people agreed to an appointment but then failed to turn up. No attempt was made to persuade anyone who clearly said they did not wish to be involved to change their mind for money. In practice, none of the offers of payment were taken up, and none of those to whom they were made took part in the study. The incentives were generous and people's reasons for turning the money down were obviously sincere and deeply felt, as with the young man who said the time had come for him to draw a line under his past and look to the future.

Overall, our best estimate is that two people were located for every one who eventually agreed to be interviewed after allowing for the three main causes of attrition: people who turned out not to be eligible for inclusion in the study (primarily because they were too young or had spent too long away from their parents as children); people who could not be contacted; and people who refused.

THE STUDY GROUP

Thirty people (sixteen men and fourteen women) were finally recruited into the study. Their ages ranged from eighteen to forty-two years for the men and sixteen to thirty-seven years for the women, with a median age for the group of twenty-seven years: over half (60 per cent) were between eighteen and thirty years old.

The subjects divide evenly into people with and people without learning difficulties. The men and women are split equally between both groups. The number of people with learning difficulties exceeded what had been planned or expected. Indeed, one of the difficulties which prolonged the fieldwork was the necessity of ensuring adequate representation of unlabelled adults. Finding grown-up children with learning difficulties was relatively much easier. This fact needs to be viewed in context. It is known that the genetic risk of parents with learning difficulties having a child with a clinically diagnosable condition is no greater than for the general population (Tymchuk, 1990b). Four specific factors aside from heredity alone seem to account for the problem. The first is an artefact of the study: adult children without learning difficulties were more likely to have moved away and less likely to be known by local service agencies or practitioners. Second, circumstantial evidence suggests that children are more likely to be removed from their parents if they do not have learning difficulties; partly because the risks to their welfare and development are seen as being that much greater and partly too because they more often present problems of control as they grow older. Consequently, fewer of them can be traced through their birth parents and more had to be excluded from the study for not having spent the greater part of their childhood with them. Third, the children of parents with learning difficulties face a high risk of developmental delay. Poverty is a major threat to their welfare. It undermines their health, their physical and intellectual development, their educational attainment, the quality of their family relationships and their emotional security. The high proportion who grow into adults with some form of learning difficulties shows what happens in the absence of effective supports designed to compensate for these deficits. Finally, the children in whom we were interested were much more likely to be excluded from mainstream school, channelled into special education and labelled as having learning difficulties because of the stigma attached to their parents.

Twenty-eight of the thirty informants had just one parent with learning difficulties, usually the mother (twenty-five cases). Although most (twenty-four) people's parents had been living together when they were born, only nine partnerships had survived death, divorce or separation, and were still intact at the start of the study. Twenty-three informants had a mother or father with learning difficulties who was still alive at the time of interview, of whom all but one remained in regular contact.

The study group included six pairs of siblings. Eighteen people came from families of three or more children; and eight people had no brothers or sisters. Eleven subjects were either married or divorced – including three women with learning difficulties – of whom all but one had children of their own. The two mothers with learning difficulties had both had their children taken into care. There was one couple in which both the husband and wife were involved in the study in their own right. Twenty-two people were unemployed at the time of interview (including all those with learning difficulties); six of the eight men without learning difficulties were in paid work. There were just three owner occupiers in the group: twenty-two people lived in council accommodation and the remainder rented privately. Thirteen people were still living with their parents of whom nine had learning difficulties. Six people with learning difficulties were living independently in their own homes, all with some paid support.

THE INTERVIEWS

Eighty-two interviews were completed with the thirty people who took part in the study. The interviews were based on the narrative method of 'life review' in which people are invited to reflect on and appraise their past experience from their standpoint in the here-and-now (Birren and Deutchman, 1991; Magee, 1988). An *aide-memoire* was used to provide a framework for the interviews and as a checklist for marking off material that had been covered, and for pinpointing topics for discussion and information needing to be collected at a subsequent session. A few direct questions were included which it was felt should be asked in the same manner of all informants. Otherwise the interviews were conducted as free-ranging conversations in which the interviewer's prompting and questioning, though disciplined by the *aide memoire*, were driven by the storyline determined by the informant.

The interviews were not intended to produce factually accurate or verifiable accounts of lives; narratives whose details would stand up to cross-checking against independent evidence or other sources of information. A distinction must be made between the stories people tell and the lives they lead. The story does not simply 'display the life' (Plummer, 1990). People reconstruct their own past in the light of their present sense of who they are. Memories constitute one of the building blocks of identity and the meanings people give to their own past are intimately bound up with the image they choose to present to others. From this point of view, people's stories about their own childhood provide a way of conceptualising the link between their upbringing and who they have become in adult life. The methodological problems of trying to establish a causal connection between family processes and later outcomes for people brought up by parents with learning difficulties are probably insurmountable. The use of narrative methods opens up the possibility of establishing a bridge through people's subjective interpretation of their own lived experience.

The fieldwork was planned on the assumption that three interviews would be required with each informant in order to cover the ground mapped out by the *aide-memoire*. The form and content of each of these interviews differed.

- The first interview was about making introductions, clarifying the purpose of the study, outlining what the interviews would be about and how the material would be used, answering any questions the person might have, assessing people's strengths and limitations as informants, finding out who's who in their family, and starting to

build up a picture of their background and their life now. The aim
was to leave as much as possible of the talking to the informant.

- The second interview placed more emphasis on the evaluative
  aspects of narrative (Kohli, 1981). As well as filling out the details of
  their life story, people were also encouraged to explore their feelings
  as a child (about, for example, their parents and grandparents, their
  schooldays, their family life, the problems they had gone through), to
  reflect on their experience of growing up, and to assess the significance of their upbringing in terms of their current situation.
  Information provided in the first interview often served as the cue for
  raising these topics.
- The third interview was used to go through the informant's story as
  recounted during the two previous sessions, make good any gaps (as
  pointed out by the interviewee or by reference to the *aide-memoire*
  material), and address the issues of representation (ensuring the story
  is true to the person) and ownership (ensuring the person shares the
  version of their life as reported). More direct questioning was often
  called for at this stage. Also people were by now usually a lot easier
  about the set-up and more trusting of the interviewer so making it
  possible to raise some sensitive issues that had been passed over in
  earlier interviews.

A full set of interviews was completed with twenty-three of the thirty
informants (four interviews were necessary in the case of one woman
with learning difficulties). A third interview was not obtained with five
people: three called a halt after two meetings ostensibly because of new
work commitments or starting college courses; one failed to turn up for
their last appointment; and another man with mental health problems
was evasive about fixing up a third meeting. A single interview only was
had with two people: in both cases it was the informant's parents who
decided to withdraw on their behalf.

The interviews were carried out in small batches of seven to eight
informants at a time in order that the interviewer could keep up with
each person's story as it unfolded and grew more detailed. Although
part of the initial fieldwork plan, such a staggered approach was in any
case made inevitable by the difficulties encountered in locating and
contacting subjects. No more than three weeks were allowed to elapse
between successive interviews in order to maintain people's interest and
commitment, and usually the gap was closer to two weeks. Almost all
(seventy-nine) of the eighty-two interviews were tape recorded with the
informant's consent and later transcribed. The one person who refused

to be recorded readily agreed to notes being taken. Two sisters asked to see the text of their story, and another man agreed to having his interviews recorded after being offered a copy of the tapes. All informants were promised a summary of the findings once the study had been finished.

A number of methods in addition to direct questioning were used to unlock people's memories, gain access to their lives, elicit information and encourage them to talk.

Photographs

Asking to see people's family photos was an effective way of finding out about family members and family relationships, bringing back the past, triggering recollections, facilitating self-reflection, stimulating conversation, focusing discussion, and easing informants into their role. Photographs are useful to the interviewer in three ways. They help to take the spotlight off the informant (who is made to feel less self-conscious and more in control). They help to legitimise the asking of questions and the interviewer's curiosity. They also have a totemic significance by providing a visual representation of the nature of people's family ties: compare, for instance, the son whose sparse collection of family photos pictured no-one outside his immediate family unit, the woman who brought out five hefty albums full of snaps of family gatherings, group holidays, celebrations and set-piece wedding portraits, and the five people who had no photographs at all of their parents.

Writing stories

Eleven people were asked to write a short story about an episode in their life of their own choosing, and seven of them delivered. The purpose was to see if people were prepared to reveal themselves through writing in ways they would not using the spoken word (Rowland *et al.*, 1990). The stories were not intended to present a complete picture or set of facts in themselves, but to open up the perspectives through which people made their own experience comprehensible and to identify topics which might become a focus for further enquiry. They also helped to verify or develop points raised in interview.

Shared interviews

Ten interviews were conducted involving two sets of brothers and sisters, a pair of sisters and a married couple in which both informants were seen at the same time. These came about for reasons of design and necessity, including the wishes and convenience of the people themselves, the impracticality of meeting them alone, and the promise of better rapport. Shared interviews brought a number of benefits. They helped to give some people the confidence to talk more freely; allowed them to spark off each other; encouraged disclosure through mutual prompting and cross-questioning; made possible verification of factual data; and provided a measure of emotional support when talking about sometimes painful events. They also helped to illuminate the effects of such variables as birth order, gender and personality on people's experiences and their resilience in the face of adversity. Bertaux (1981) says that 'a good life story is one in which the interviewee *takes over the control of the interview situation*' (italics in original). Such an occurrence implies a measure of self-assurance and fluency rarely encountered among most informants, least of all those with learning difficulties. However, shared interviews did tend to empower informants by making them feel less vulnerable to the interviewer's attention.

Switching off the tape recorder

Putting aside the tape recorder for a spell during an interview was often a useful gambit, especially in the case of more reserved informants. Doing so served a variety of purposes: to relax the informant; to check whether the recorder was having an inhibiting effect; to mark the shift to a new and perhaps sensitive topic; and to give both parties a breather. Switching off made it possible to see if the person felt any easier about talking, and helped to 'break the ice' on a new topic before recording was started again. Issues that might require careful handling could be approached in an 'off-the record' fashion. Also, though rarely acknowledged in the literature, the practice of recording puts a lot of strain on the interviewer, who is constantly aware of being 'on air' and playing to an audience (including the transcriber and any research colleagues). This knowledge exerts a subliminal pressure to say the right thing, keep the conversation flowing, stick to the point, phrase the questions appropriately, attend to leads and generally deliver a good performance. Switching off may be done several times during an interview for any number of these reasons.

ISSUES FOR NARRATIVE RESEARCH

People organise their experience and their memory mainly in the form of narrative (Bruner, 1991). This study set out to make use of this human capacity for 'storying' experience in order to capture something of what it means to be brought up by parents with learning difficulties. Stories invite the listener 'to imagine, and in imagining to experience, the worlds created in the words' (Scheppele, 1989). Connelly and Clandinin (1990), for instance, suggest that a good story is one that can be lived vicariously by others. Our aim was to harness the power of narrative in order to depict the lives of our subjects at the level of feeling as well as understanding. The success of this venture obviously depended on the responsiveness of our informants. A number of inhibiting factors limited some people's ability to talk freely.

Inarticulateness

Inarticulateness refers to an inability to communicate fluently in words: an inability that goes beyond mere shyness, anxiety or reserve. It originates with restricted language skills, but is generally overlaid by other factors such as lack of self-esteem, learned habits of compliance, loneliness and the experience of social exclusion. Although more commonly encountered among our informants with learning difficulties, it was not confined to them. Inarticulateness does not present an insuperable barrier to people telling their story (see chapter 3). However, it does have implications for the role of the interviewer (who must expect to work harder) and for the way stories are turned into text (where the hand of the editor will be more apparent). Sometimes there was simply not enough direct speech to render a person's story in their own words. But third-person accounts of lives usually lose the immediacy and authenticity of the subject's own voice. In order to ensure that the important emotional dimension of narrative is not lost with inarticulate subjects, researchers must be prepared to experiment with methods of reporting that allow more scope for the play of what George Eliot called 'the veracious imagination', including the fictional form (Booth, 1995; Clough, 1996).

Temporality

Talking about experience, as Clandinin and Connelly (1994) point out, 'is to talk temporally'. Time is what holds a life story together and gives it both structure and meaning. The self as narrator, however, exists only in the present. Language is necessary in order to abstract the self into the past (or an anticipated future). It is only through language that the self has a sense of itself in the past. For people with restricted language skills, like some of those with learning difficulties in our study, the inability to objectify the self found its expression in a strong present orientation and a concrete frame of reference that countermanded the tick-tock essentials of good storytelling.

The reticence of young people

Many of the younger adults in our study struggled to find a voice. Such reticence did not come about because they were unable to express themselves. They were just not sure they had anything worth saying. Lack of confidence in the validity of one's own experience is a characteristic of youth. People must first know what they know before they can begin to narrate their own stories. Informants who had less to say tended to be younger people (with or without learning difficulties) whose lives were still closely bound up with their parents or who, irrespective of age, had not yet fully negotiated the transition into adulthood. Dickerson and Zimmerman (1993) have conceived adolescence as a time when young people are living stories in which they are the protagonist rather than the narrator. Building on this insight, it may be that establishing an identity of one's own is a prerequisite for carrying off the role of narrator in the story of one's life.

Poor recall

Some people seemed to have scant memories of their childhood. Why this should be is not immediately apparent although Bruner (1987) provides a possible clue. He suggests that storytelling provides recipes for structuring experience itself and for laying down routes into memory. The stories that constitute children and young people's lives are usually told for them by others (Zimmerman and Dickerson, 1994). Autobiographical memories of childhood come from the sharing of such stories, primarily between parents and children. It is possible that parents with learning difficulties engage in less 'memory talk' of this kind with their children so limiting what their children know about their own past. The absence of family photographs may serve as one clue that such a store of remembering has not been laid down. People who lack fully storied lives may not be able to access their own experience through memory or know they have a story to tell.

Interview cuckoos

The researcher was not always able to control who was present during an interview. Aside from the shared interviews, where two informants were seen together, twelve interviews involving ten people were conducted with someone else in the room for all or part of the time. Usually this was a parent, spouse or partner, although cuckoos also included a friend and various practitioners. Family members were present for two of the interviews with two people; in all other cases supernumeraries were there for only one of the three sessions. The other person was always present on the express wish of the informant. Although better avoided if possible, having an informed other occasionally sit in on an interview was not always a bad thing, especially given the problems of reticence and poor recall mentioned above. Parents in particular were sometimes useful for triggering early memories or raising issues that could be explored later when the subject was next seen alone. The essential flexibility of the narrative method provides a check against possible bias from this source: the same material can always be revisited at a later date, or a further interview can be added to make good one spoiled.

'Writing about the past,' Steedman (1990) says, 'must always be done out of a set of current preoccupations.' Here the past in question is the childhood of our now-adult subjects. The preoccupations we bring to our topic are a zeal for narrative research and an interest in parenting by people with learning difficulties. In this chapter we have shown how these strands were brought together in this study. The next chapter looks more closely at the challenge of conducting narrative research with inarticulate subjects.

Chapter 3

Talking with Danny Avebury

People with learning difficulties present the narrative researcher with a number of challenges among which three stand out as particularly important. None of these are unique to their label; they are also encountered with other informants. Equally, they may well arise in prospect more than in practice. But researchers should at least be prepared for them before they enter the field.

The first of these problems is *unresponsiveness*: a limited ability to answer some types of question. In a series of studies designed to test the efficacy of different question formats with respondents who have learning difficulties, Sigelman and her colleagues (Sigelman *et al.*, 1981a; Sigelman *et al.*, 1982; Sigelman *et al.*, 1981b) found that open-ended questions received the poorest response. Few respondents could answer them adequately and those who could provided relatively little information. Biklen and Moseley (1988) likewise 'suggest avoiding open-ended questions'. Yet in narrative research it is generally agreed that interviews should be 'open and fluid' in order to enable the subject 'to take the lead' (Plummer, 1983). Contrary to Thompson's observation (1981) that most material is normally 'narrated independently of direct questions', the lack of responsiveness to open-ended questioning by informants with learning difficulties usually requires the researcher to adopt a more direct style of interviewing.

The second problem is characterised by a *concrete frame of reference* that leads to difficulties in generalising from experience and thinking in abstract terms. According to Labov and Waletzky (1967), narratives have both a referential and an evaluative function (Kohli, 1981). The referential function involves reconstructing past events in some sort of chronological order. The evaluative function involves relating these past events to the present: reconstructing the meaning of the past from a position in the here-and-now in order to give meaning to the present

(Bertaux-Wiame, 1981). The concrete frame of reference typical of many people with learning difficulties cramps their capacity for looking back on their own past with the sort of reflexivity the evaluative function demands. Consequently it is often hard to establish the significance of past events in people's lives. While Spradley (1979) has pointed out that people who are overly abstract are often less useful as informants, people with learning difficulties present a challenge for precisely the opposite reasons.

Third come *problems with time* as revealed by a strong present orientation and difficulties with dates and numbers. These problems are only partly a consequence of not knowing how to tell the time or use a calendar. They are also indicative of lives which lack many of the milestones people use to order their past – such as examinations, the driving test, first car, starting work, setting up home, job changes, promotions, marriage, parenthood etc. – and many of the props – trophies, certificates, photo albums, scrap books, possessions – people use for marking the passage of time. Flynn (1986) advises that questions about time and frequency are best avoided when interviewing people with learning difficulties (Atkinson, 1988). Biklen and Moseley (1988) similarly report that their 'informants often confused time sequences and settings'. While ways can often be found around some of these problems (Booth and Booth, 1994a), they do put limits on the important referential function of narrative which is essentially a story in time.

Plummer (1983) observes that good informants 'should be fairly articulate, able to verbalise and have "a good story to tell"'. For the reasons outlined above, informants with learning difficulties who satisfy these criteria are likely to prove the exception rather than the rule. However, this fact alone should not be seen as an excuse for discounting the usefulness of narrative methods. Fluency is not the only key to communication. Silence may be as telling as talk. When using narrative methods with people who have learning difficulties, researchers must learn to read the spaces between the words. Our aim in this chapter is to show what this means in practical terms. Let us begin with a story.

DANNY AVEBURY'S STORY

Danny Avebury is twenty years old and has learning difficulties. He is the eldest of four children and lives with his parents on a small council estate. The family has always lived in the same house. Danny likes where he lives; the neighbours are friendly, he says. They have no telephone, and no car as neither of his parents drive. Both his mother and father have learning difficulties. Two younger sisters still live at home and attend special school; Danny's nineteen-year-old brother, Bob, has moved out to live with his girlfriend. Bob has a car but Danny hasn't seen him since he left home. Danny, his parents and his brother are all unemployed. When Danny left special school at sixteen, he enrolled at a further education college to study maths, English and computer work. Two days a week he does voluntary work on a community farm and one morning he goes with the gardening group from college to trim hedges and cut the lawn at an old people's home.

Danny is tall and slim with black hair which has recently been cut from shoulder length. His mum cuts his hair. He has a friendly manner and smiles frequently. He wears a baseball cap and the casual clothes of his generation although they are a bit on the large size. He usually carries with him a large holdall bag for his books and personal stereo. He smokes.

Out of college Danny spends most of his time at home watching television. His favourite programmes are 'Home and Away' and football matches. He rarely goes to bed before one o'clock as he likes to watch the late night films. He also enjoys listening to local radio and tapes on his stereo; his favourite singers are Meatloaf and Belinda Carlisle and he has posters of Madonna on his bedroom wall. Occasionally he goes shopping with his mum, or accompanies his parents to the local pub. He doesn't belong to any clubs and has never been to the cinema. When he goes out in an evening, it is to sit on his front wall and talk to his friends in the neighbourhood. They are all much younger than him. There is a student at college whom he would like to get to know better, perhaps one day even to call his girlfriend, but at present he sees her only from a distance.

He has friends at college but doesn't see them outside. He says his parents stop him going out. He only remembers going on holiday once, to Cleethorpes, and that was with college. He has never been on holiday with his parents. His mum and dad have no regular friends whom they visit or who come to see them.

At home Danny says his mum does most of the jobs around the house, including the shopping. His dad does 'nowt': just sits around most of the time, although occasionally he will do some gardening. Danny washes the pots for his mum, and sometimes helps his dad in the garden, but his main job is to look after the family pets – a budgerigar, a cat, eighteen tropical fish, two rabbits and a ferret. He found the ferret. When Danny leaves college he would like to work with animals.

Danny's one freedom is his racer bike on which he takes himself off to the park for a ride – always on his own and only during the daytime.

This Christmas he has asked for rollerblades like his friend Adam's.

As a child, Danny used to be collected from home by a special bus. Today he catches two buses to college. He enjoyed his school days and liked his teachers. He had friends at school but never played with his brother who went to a different school and mixed with a different crowd. His mum and dad have always taken an interest in his education. They regularly attended parents' evenings at his special school and recently were at college to see him presented with a certificate for his achievements.

Danny is unable to remember much at all about his childhood, not even when his sisters were born. He cannot remember ever seeing his grandparents nor any other relatives but, he says, he has never felt lonely. The one incident from the past he does remember well is when he went out with his brother and stole a car. Danny was the passenger. The police came to see his parents and gave him a stern warning. It has never happened again. Although his brother has now left home, Danny is still watched very closely by his parents.

He wishes he could make more decisions for himself, like choosing to go out at night or to keep his hair long. His sister once tied his hair back in a pony tail, and he rather liked it that way, but his mother decided he should have it cut short. Danny sometimes has arguments with his parents, especially about going out, but on the whole they get on all right. He feels they are a close family. He loves his mum and dad.

THE ORIGINS OF DANNY'S STORY

Danny Avebury was one of the people who took part in our study. We have chosen to recount his story because Danny presents an extreme example of the general problem of inarticulateness that narrative researchers might expect to encounter – usually in a less severe form – when interviewing people with learning difficulties. As such, his story and the interviews from which it has been put together merit closer analysis for two reasons.

First, they demonstrate that narrative research is not fatally compromised by Baron's (1991) paradox: that those who most need to have their stories heard may be least able to tell them. It is possible to use narrative methods to give a voice to people who lack words, and to gain a measure of access to the lives of even the most inarticulate and unresponsive informants. They may yield a much poorer harvest of material than would be obtained from studies involving better informants, but enough nonetheless to make the effort worthwhile in a literature that is still largely 'void of the experience it would presumably portray' (Whittemore *et al.*, 1986). Second, Danny's story contains general lessons for narrative researchers which challenge the view that the problems of interviewing inarticulate subjects arise from their own limitations.

Danny Avebury was chronically short of words. He would only speak when spoken to, and then as little as possible. During three interviews running to almost two and a half hours of recorded conversation he uttered only ten complete sentences, including four 'don't knows' and a 'can't remember'. His longest sentence was made up of five words. His fullest reply came to a question about his pets when he said he had 'a rabbit an' all, and a ferret'. Otherwise, his responses to three out of every four questions consisted of a single word only.

There is no reason to suppose that Danny's reticence was his way of saying he did not wish to be interviewed. He always greeted the researcher with a smile and a friendly hello. He willingly agreed to the second and third interviews. He never failed to turn up. Indeed, on one occasion he rang to say that he had a dental appointment and might not make it back to college in time, but was there on the day as arranged.

In an effort to find some way of drawing him out, an informal group discussion was arranged with his tutorial class at college. We wondered if Danny might be a bit more forthcoming given the support and example of his peers. The group comprised nine students of whom five had learning difficulties and four were catching up on their education. They had all known each other for some time. Conversation was guided around commonplace issues such as what people liked doing best at college, what they liked doing in their spare time, what jobs they did around the home, what they would like to do when they leave college, and so on. Danny was even quieter than usual. In an hour's recorded discussion he spoke just forty words, and then only in response to direct questions put to him. Observation of him with his tutors confirmed the reactive nature of his conversation and the monosyllabic quality of his speech. Danny, we concluded, just didn't have much talk in him.

THE MAKING OF A NARRATIVE

In narrative research, according to Thompson (1981), it is 'normal for much of the material in the interview to be narrated independently of direct questions'. The reverse is more likely to be true in the case of inarticulate subjects. Danny Avebury only replied to direct questions, and then not always. This puts more onus on the skill of the researcher who must not only work harder (by having to ask more questions and probe more fully to elicit information) but also pay more regard to the form of the questions, the sort of language used, and the conduct of the interview. Part of the problem here is that 'we have very few ways of conversing with persons who are not as smart as we are' (Biklen and Moseley, 1988). Too often these ways involve talking down to people as if their lack of words denotes a lack of comprehension. The researcher must establish a level of communication that facilitates rapport without making people feel inadequate. Our experience is that even the most inarticulate people generally discern a great deal more than their conversation reveals. We have found it important to begin interviews without any fixed assumptions about people's ability to understand what was being asked of them. Their abilities have to be tested.

At the same time as coaxing conversation out of people the researcher is also having to explore the efficacy of different modes of questioning in an effort to find ways of helping them respond. Tremblay (1957) has described this technique as 'self-developing' in that the researcher must refine the 'interviewing method during the course of a session, or through repeated contacts, as the amount of knowledge about the problem increases and as the ability of the informant is fully revealed'. Looking more closely at Danny's transcripts provides a useful window on this process at work.

Danny was not able to cope with open-ended questions. Any form of question that did not lend itself to a one-word reply was usually met with silence:

Int: Can you try and think back to when you were a small child. What is the very first thing you can remember?

DA: (*Long silence*)

Int: Is there any particular thing you remember . . . that stands out in your mind? It might be a good thing, it might be a bad thing.

DA: (*Very long silence*)

Int: Nothing coming to you?

DA: No.

These silences were not all of a kind: they were laden with at least four possible meanings. They might indicate that Danny had not understood the question or that he could not articulate the answer or that he wanted to avoid answering without actually lying or that he did not know the answer. The skill of the interviewer lies in detecting which of these possibilities applies in each instance and, therefore, in deciding how to proceed. In the case of the first two, the question might be rephrased and put again, usually in a simpler form. In the third instance, some less threatening way of approaching the topic needs to be found. In the latter case, the line of questioning might best be given up and a fresh topic broached.

A useful strategy in rephrasing questions was to break them down into simple parts asking for a yes/no response or a similar one-word answer:

Int: I want to get a picture of your mum and dad in my head. How would you describe them? How would you describe your mum for a start?

DA: (*Long silence*)

Int: What's she look like?

DA: (*Long silence*)

Int: Do you think you look like your mum or your dad?

DA: (*Silence*)

Int: Can't you say that?

DA: No.

Int: You don't know?

DA: No.

Int: And you can't describe her – is she tall?

DA: No, small.

Int: Is she dark or has she got grey hair now or is she. . . . What colour's her hair?

DA: Brown.

Int: Does she wear glasses?

DA: Yes.

Int: What about your dad? Is he small?

DA: No.

Again the open-ended question failed to elicit any information at all; its purpose is primarily to signal a change of topic and to mark out what the interviewer would like to talk about next. Note also that Danny says he cannot answer the first direct question although the easy option for him would have been to feed the interviewer by making up a reply. He seeks to answer truthfully or remains silent. (Evidence that he understood the question came later in the interview when he said he thought his sisters looked like their mum.) As the extract also demonstrates, acquiescence – the tendency to respond affirmatively regardless of the question – was not one of his traits. He was prepared to say no. This enabled the interviewer to use leading questions ('Is she tall?', 'Is he small?') as a means of probing for information that Danny would not volunteer himself. The problem with an inarticulate informant like Danny is that he does not provide any clues about what the interviewer should be asking: unlike more fluent subjects whose responses generally contain the seeds of the next question. The only practical option is to offer up a menu of suggestions with which he can either agree or disagree. The following extract from the transcripts illustrates the approach:

Int: Can you remember what toys you used to have . . . when you were small? Any toys that you used to like?
DA: (*Long silence*) No.
Int: Did you use to have toys at Christmas . . . and on your birthday?
DA: (*Long silence*)
Int: Were you given presents?
DA: (*Long silence*)
Int: You can't remember?
DA: Can't remember.
Int: What about your last birthday? What did you have on your birthday this year?
DA: I don't know.
Int: Is it that you can't remember or that you didn't have anything? . . . It doesn't matter what you say.
DA: (*Long silence*)
Int: Perhaps your family doesn't buy each other presents on their birthdays? Do they?
DA: No. . . . No.

The silences in this sequence were not empty of meaning. Danny was made a little uneasy by the topic, as if embarrassed for his family, but after trying to avoid a reply his basic honesty (and his lack of words) prevented him from giving a less than truthful response when the interviewer finally hit on the right question. By the gradual *elimination of alternatives* it is possible to piece together a story bit by bit. Equally, by the *progressive adaptation* of questions it is usually possible to find a formula that will trigger a response. Once again, this entails listening to the silences in order to detect whether the question needs putting in a different way, whether the topic needs approaching from a different tack, or whether the respondent really has nothing more to say on the subject. As the following vignette shows, direct questions alone did not always bring a reply if they outstripped Danny's comprehension:

Int: I know this is very difficult to think about, but if you ever did in the future . . . if you ever became a parent, and you had children (*Danny laughs*), do you think you would do things differently for your children than your mum and dad have done for you?

DA: (*Long silence*)

Int: Do you think you would treat them any differently?

DA: (*Long silence*)

Int: In some ways, it's a round about question that's really asking do you think your mum and dad should have treated you any differently?

DA: (*Long silence*)

Int: Is there anything you wish they'd done for you that they haven't done?

DA: No.

Int: So if you had some children you'd treat them exactly the same as your mum and dad have treated you?

DA: Yes.

Int: That's what you're saying?

DA: Yes.

What Biklen and Moseley (1988) have called this strategy of 'successive approximations' provides a grounded approach to understanding something of the subjective world of inarticulate subjects while raising two attendant dangers. Because the researcher has to do most of the pedalling, there is an ever-present risk of the interview becoming more like an interrogation. People with few words cannot easily defend themselves against unwelcome or intrusive questioning. Once again the researcher must heed the sounds of silence for those unspoken signals by which an informant indicates that enough is enough. A second danger of the strategy is that the framework within which information is obtained comes to reflect the researcher's concerns rather than the informant's own view of his or her life. There is a sense in which this is part of the price that must be paid for getting any material from inarticulate subjects. By the nature of things, their interviews rarely assume the character of a true dialogue. People who are able to express themselves easily give direction to the interview by what they say. With people who are not talkative the researcher has to be more attentive to what goes unsaid, and to learn to distinguish between an expressive silence (waiting to be broken) and a closed silence (waiting to be passed over).

There are no easy rules for distinguishing these two types of silence, except that the researcher should not give up too quickly. The clues are usually personal and idiosyncratic, and are picked up only by getting to know the informant. For this reason, interviews with inarticulate subjects should normally be spread over several sessions, and where possible supplemented by time spent with the person in other settings and situations. In Danny's case, he often implicitly invited the interviewer to probe more carefully by smiling or laughing, remaining quiet and still, or maintaining direct eye contact. Equally, he indicated his discomfort and desire to move on to some other topic by, for example, shifting around in his seat, fiddling with his watch or his clothes, or looking away. The following passage shows the interviewer responding in turn to both kinds of silence:

Int: Do you have any close friends, anybody that you see quite a lot?
DA: (*Long pause*) No.
Int: You don't have a girlfriend?
DA: (*Expressive silence*)
Int: Do you? That's not a no there. You've got somebody you'd like to call your girlfriend?
DA: Yes.
Int: What's her name?
DA: (*Closed silence*)
Int: I won't embarrass you. But you would like to get a bit closer to her?
DA: Yes.

In the first instance, Danny's demeanour indicated there was something he wanted to say and the interviewer sensed that the silence was not a barrier to further exploration of the topic. On the second occasion, the interviewer quickly perceived that she had overstepped the mark and withdrew.

Two aspects of the process of piecing together a person's story by the elimination of alternatives deserve emphasis. First, it opens up the possibility of developing a narrative by *creative guesswork*. Different story-lines may be tried out with the informant until an admissible version is established – in much the same way as a police identikit picture is assembled. Take the following example:

Int: Have you had any trouble with the police?
DA: (*Looks sheepish and doesn't answer*)
Int: Looks like there might have been a bit of bother at some time. What was that?

DA: (*Silence*)

Int: Was that you or your brother? This is strictly confidential. It's not going to go anywhere.

DA: (*Laughs*)

Int: I'm not going to tell anybody else. It's just to get a feeling of the sort of life you've had. You've had a bit of trouble with the police?

DA: Yes

Int: What, you?

DA: Both of us.

Int: What happened? . . . What were you doing?

DA: (Silence)

Int: Did they just come round and have a word with your mum and dad?

DA: Yes.

Int: What, just to warn you was it?

DA: Yes. (*Laughs*)

Int: Can you tell me about it, because it sounds as if it's something in the past now. What had happened?

DA: (*Silence*)

Int: Had you been messing around and sort of throwing things or spraying things or . . . ?

DA: (*Silence*)

Int: No? It's none of those, is it?

DA: No.

Int: Was it you and Bob together doing it?

DA: Yes.

Int: Were you nicking cars?

DA: Yes.

Int: So it was Bob who was driving?

DA: Yes.

Int: And you were passenger, were you?

DA: Yes. (*Laughs*)

Int: How many cars did you nick then?

DA: One.

Int: Just the one?

DA: Yes.

This technique is crucially dependent on the veracity of the informant. It will not work unless he or she can be trusted to reject a false narrative hypothesis. Danny had already established himself as a truthful lad. His inability to put himself into hypothetical situations stripped him of the capacity to deceive. His only alternative to telling the truth was to remain silent. When he spoke he meant what he said. Secure in this knowledge, it was possible for the interviewer to suggest likely scenarios ('Were you nicking cars?') in order to weave a story from the resulting yeses and noes. This method does not easily square with standard text-book guidance on good interviewing practice. It can be seen as putting words into the mouths of informants. Our position is that the challenge of interviewing inarticulate subjects calls for unorthodox methods. The only way of collecting their stories may be to loan them the words.

A second point to note about this approach is that stories also evolve in the absence of concrete information. Ruling things out can be as revealing as a wealth of detail. When Danny says that he doesn't go out with friends, doesn't go out in an evening, doesn't belong to any clubs, has never been to a football match, has never been on holiday with his mum and dad, has never been on any school trips, doesn't receive birthday presents, and that neither his father nor his mother nor his brother have a job, he evokes a childhood corroded by poverty and bounded by narrow horizons without having need of any rhetorical skills. Stories can emerge in a succession of noes to direct questions about everyday personal experience.

This leads to a final point. It is possible for people to communicate a story in one-word answers. Even single words can leave a big wash. Denzin (1989) may be right when he argues that lives are available to us only in words, but we must avoid the mistake of assuming that we cannot access the lives of people who have difficulty stringing them together. The following edited extract from Danny's interviews shows why:

Int: What do you do on a Monday?
DA: Farm.
Int: What's the farm? It's not here . . . whereabouts is that?
DA: No. Bretton.
Int: What do you do up there?
DA: Planting.
    . . .
Int: What do you think you'll do when you leave here then? Have you thought?
DA: No.
Int: What would you like to do?
DA: On a farm. Hartshead Farm.

Int: What, with animals though?
DA: Yes.

These same questions put to someone who was more forthcoming might have been expected to produce more quotable material. Yet Danny's close-mouthed responses, taken with what he said elsewhere in the interviews, provide their own eloquent picture of a lonely young man, with no realistic hope of a job, putting up with a college placement doing gardening that he doesn't really enjoy while dreaming of working with animals, like the pets he looks after at home.

Danny's poor self-expression may not prevent him from telling his story, but it does have implications for the way it is turned into text. There is insufficient continuous speech in the interviews to present the story in Danny's own words. This makes it necessary for the researcher as editor to play a fuller part in reconstituting the transcripts as narrative. The story as told above has been cast as a third-person account. While true to the material it loses the authenticity of the subject's own voice. Certainly, the issue of representation – who is doing the talking and how accurately the text reflects the data – assumes a particular importance with inarticulate subjects (see chapter 7).

CONCLUSIONS

Danny Avebury's story presents meagre pickings for almost two and a half hours of interview time. A Studs Terkel or Tony Parker would not make a living out of the Danny Aveburys of the world. Yet for all its lack of narrative depth or richness Danny's story is revealing as one of a type. It properly belongs to a class of stories about the problems that young people with learning difficulties have in negotiating the transition to adulthood. The drift is in the detail. Danny, at twenty years old, is not allowed out at nights. He spends his evenings sitting on the garden wall talking to the younger children in the neighbourhood or watching television by himself. He enjoys riding his racer bike on his own in the park, and would like a pair of rollerblades for Christmas. He sometimes goes to the pub with his mum and dad. His mum cuts his hair, and not how he likes. He has never had a girlfriend. He would like more say in making his own decisions. These particulars of Danny's story are a manifestation of a more general theme – the adult-as-child – which similarly finds expression in the accounts of others like him. Put alongside these other stories, Danny's narrative has a valuable role to play in making this abstract theme more tangible in personal terms (Abrams,

1991). It also illustrates the truth of Biklen and Moseley's (1988) dictum that, 'Nothing is trivial to qualitative researchers'. The small particulars and happenings that Danny so sparingly relates assume a symbolic meaning as part of a story shared with others.

There is another reason too for paying attention to Danny Avebury. Too often the problems of interviewing inarticulate subjects are seen in terms of their deficits rather than the limitations of our methods. Such a 'deficit model' of informant response is rooted in a view of disability as a problem of the individual. It serves to legitimate the exclusion of, for example, people with learning difficulties from a participatory role in narrative research in ways that mirror their exclusion from the wider society. The emphasis of research should be on overcoming the barriers that impede the involvement of inarticulate subjects instead of highlighting the difficulties they present. Conventional research methods can create obstacles for inarticulate subjects in terms of the demands they make on their inclusion. The lesson to be drawn from Danny's story is that researchers should attend more to their own deficiencies than to the limitations of their informants.

It is too easy as a narrative researcher not to bother with people like Danny; to argue that the investment is not worth the return just because it does not generate good text. There is a danger of allowing ourselves to be drawn by the tempo of our times into a kind of 'fast research' with a premium on quick results. Against this background, it is important to remember the virtues of an older, anthropological tradition which recognised that the task of learning to communicate with subjects takes a long time. Narrative researchers must go back to such basics in order to ensure that their scholarship does not continue to silence the stories of people like Danny Avebury.

Chapter 4

What became of the children we used to be

In this chapter we begin the task of trying to make sense of how the now-adult children in our study fared growing up in a family headed by at least one parent with learning difficulties, and at the kind of lives they had made for themselves. Trying to capture lives 'in the round' is not an easy task. The data generated by our study come in the form of stories. They cannot easily be squeezed into tables or plotted on graphs. Words rather than numbers are the raw material of narrative research, and they are not so amenable to aggregation. A proper starting point is to listen to some stories as told.

BONNIE CRAVEN

Bonnie Craven is thirty-three years old and lives with her mother and younger sister, Susie, on a council estate in a busy mining village. All three have learning difficulties. Her father died a few years ago and since then the family has received support from the Community Learning Disabilities Team. Bonnie and her sister are both regular churchgoers: 'The dress what I got christened in, it were made off my mam's wedding dress.' She recalls how they were made to go to Sunday School 'because if you didn't they used to come looking for you'.

Bonnie is a tall woman, slightly overweight, with a smiling, attractive face. She has pale auburn, wavy hair, tied up with a red ribbon. Bonnie chose to be interviewed in a quiet room at the local town hall rather than at home where she feared she might lack the privacy to speak candidly. She arrived wearing a turquoise jumper, white beads, black stretch leggings and high heels. Her initial shyness vanished almost immediately and she needed little prompting to talk.

When Bonnie was born her family lived in a large city but soon after they moved out to the village where she now lives. They lived with her father's parents until they were allocated their own council tenancy. Bonnie still lives in the same house. Her father was a crane driver and her mother used to work at a sweet-making factory before she married. Her father was a handyman around the house, making clothes for all the family on an automatic knitting machine. He was also an amateur photographer and Bonnie remembers as a teenager helping him develop his own films.

Bonnie attended a special school 'because I were slow at learning'. When she left, at sixteen, she went to a further education college to take cooking and dressmaking. After her courses had finished, she stayed at home for a while. 'I asked our Susie if there were somewhere I could go because I were getting bored. And our Susie asked her community nurse and she came to see me.'

At the moment, on a Monday and Friday, she is learning some more maths and improving her writing skills at a centre. Tuesdays she attends another centre: 'We play badminton, table tennis, there's pool and there's board games.' On Wednesdays she usually does the washing or other housework at home. She goes horse riding on Thursdays when there are sessions for disabled people. Saturdays are spent cleaning the silver in her local church. And Sundays, after church, 'I don't do much. We have us dinners and if it's a nice day we go a walk.'

School for Bonnie was a mixed experience. She 'used to get bullied a lot . . . when we were outside at playtime. I weren't right good at mixing.' She found protection by sticking close to the teacher on duty in the play-ground. The headmaster was particularly strict and she herself had been punished at times with both the slipper and the cane. However she used to enjoy the school trips, and once went on a week's holiday with the school. She also remembers, with a smile, her parents coming up to school on open evenings and sports days: 'I used to love it when they used to walk through door.' She learned to read and write, and can manage money. Bonnie remembers her parents talking to the headmaster about her going to the local comprehensive school: 'He said, "I won't allow Bonnie to go to Keswick School because they're too rough", and I got sent to Seaton at Crompton.' She had wanted to go to Keswick.

When Bonnie was a child her mum and dad shared the domestic chores, especially the cooking and shopping, although her father was always in charge of the money side of things. He would also watch over Bonnie's mum when she did the cooking: 'He were really good to my mam. He used to keep an eye on her.' Her grandparents often used to babysit if her parents went out and most days they would have Bonnie and her sister after school and give them their tea: 'My grandma used to play with us and she used to play piano and that. She wasn't boring, she used to be right entertaining. We were very close, me and my grandma.'

As Bonnie grew older she rather liked her parents to go out so that she could be by herself and listen to her records:

> Every time my mam went out with my dad, they always fetched us summat back from pub, packet of crisps and pop. Sometimes it used to be cheese biscuits. When I got older they started fetching me drinks and that, like Babychams.

When her dad was still alive, Bonnie's favourite meal was meat stew and Yorkshire pudding. Today she mostly makes do with pre-cooked, convenience meals although, she says, 'I started making fruit salad, fresh fruit salad. My mam loves it.' Sometimes, on a Sunday, her mum will cook a chicken or chops – but Bonnie has to keep a check on her, just like her dad did.

The whole family regularly went to places such as Bridlington, Scarborough and Skegness for their holidays: 'My grandma and granddad used to come with us.' Bonnie's grandma regularly took her shopping and Bonnie often accompanied her father too when he went out: 'I used to go all over with him.' She can't remember going anywhere with her mum on her own. She had a few close, childhood friends: 'We used to play outside a lot. We used to play games on street, hide and seek and all them.' As a teenager she had been a member of the local youth club where she liked playing table tennis and badminton. Bonnie can only cite one close friend that she has now – her neighbour across the road who has spina bifida. They have known each other since they were little girls. She has friends at the centre, but no-one visits her at home. Bonnie likes watching television and hires videos of musicals and back episodes of TV serials such as 'Neighbours' and 'Coronation Street'. Occasionally she does some embroidery.

Bonnie only remembers being ill with measles as a child and had no serious accidents. One incident, though, does stick in her mind.

> Once, my mam were out and – you know them things you shake up with snow? – Mam used to have a big one, and it was on top of piano, and I reached to get it down and I dropped it, and it all smashed all over. I ran upstairs and I slipped, because we had oil cloth then, and carpet, and I went right under bed and banged my head, cut it open. My dad ran upstairs, got me, carried me downstairs, and he got on phone to doctor. My dad took me to hospital, I

remember that, and there were all kids on street looking, watching. I went to hospital and they put stitches in and I were roaring.

There was no shortage of toys as a child: 'I remember one Christmas, I woke up, there were presents all round my bed. I remember because I can still see them.' While Bonnie had a lot of loving attention from her father she only once remembers receiving a hug from her mother. Nor did she ever see her parents hug each other – although, then again, they didn't quarrel much either.

Bonnie has spent a long time trying to come to terms with some of her father's behaviour. 'I've had some good life and I've some bad life an' all. . . . used to have bad times with my dad. He used to be cruel.' Mostly he was a loving father who 'used to be nice, lovely with me', but on Sundays, after he had been to the pub, he often turned on her violently, hitting her over the head with his hand. 'I didn't know what it were for, I didn't know. I don't think I were doing nowt. I used to get it a lot.' Bonnie told her best friend over the road and confided in her local vicar, whom she knew very well, but she told him not to do anything. 'Didn't want my dad to get into trouble. Don't want that, be more upsetting, I think.' Her father's cruelty, in other ways so out of char-acter, had gone on for a few years and darkened her memory of him. Now that he was dead she felt she would never really know why he had singled her out for such punishment.

Bonnie says she used to 'get it too when I were younger with my mam'. But that was different. When you're naughty and won't do as you're told you expect to get into bother. She and her sister would be sent to their bedrooms if they misbehaved: 'They said you're going to bed without no tea, you're having no lemon curd. I used to love that lemon curd, me.'

Bonnie remembers her dad waiting up for her once when she came back late with a friend from an Osmonds' concert in Manchester. He looked after her like that. But she also recalls having been sexually molested by a friend of her father's who touched her – 'not just me, it were our Susie an' all' – in ways she did not like when she was about nine years old.

It were somebody called Bob, come to our house. He used to come and see my dad. Used to come on trips with us, an' all. My dad used to keep an eye on him all time. My granddad used to say, 'Keep an eye on them lasses.'

Bonnie told her father about this man. 'He stopped, yes.'

Her father's parents lived close by and helped them out in all sorts of practical ways. Bonnie was very close to them:

> My granddad once made a dolls' house and it used to light up, and he used to have it in front of window and people used to pass and look at it. My grandma tells me things about her life: about war and all stuff like that. I'm interested when they talk to me about it all.

An aunt and uncle too were often around and on hand when needed. Both Grandma and Granddad Craven are now dead and Bonnie wishes there was someone to help manage the house and garden. Her mother's parents are now infirm and her uncle has died: 'We don't see hardly nobody now.'

After her father died Bonnie's mother found it very hard to manage: 'I think she's feeling lost without him. You know how some people talk. . . . They meet friends – like other women – talk and go out. My mam doesn't do that.' Bonnie remembers the day her father died very clearly.

> I were coming downstairs, my mam came to bottom. She says, 'I'm going to hospital.' She says, 'Your dad's right poorly today.' And I goes, 'Oh no.' I knew what were going to happen, me. I had this right strange feeling. My Auntie Anne come and Uncle Bill and I could tell summat were up because they weren't laughing. They sat me down and told me. I just busted out crying. I didn't know where I was. I lost use of myself.

Since her husband's death, Bonnie's mother has almost become a recluse. She doesn't like leaving the house, not even to accompany Bonnie and her sister when they go out for a drink to the local pub.

Bonnie is beginning to feel she has a bit too much to do in the house, as most of the jobs fall on her. She began to help with the housework while still at school: 'I remember starting cleaning up. My mam and dad went out and I were left in house on my own. That's when I first started cleaning up.' Now she doesn't enjoy it like she did. 'I'm in need of some help,' she says, especially with their large garden. 'We're not good at that.' The local vicar said he would get someone to cut their grass 'but I think he's forgot since then'.

Bonnie has never had a boyfriend. She 'used to dance with them and that, used to like lads, yes, used to like them. I like them for a friend to talk to, and I like teasing them an' all, just like having big brothers. But,' she muses, it's 'not easy to get one.'

Looking to the future, Bonnie would like a little house for herself.

Her sister will shortly be moving into a group home. Just now, however, Bonnie prefers to look after her mother. 'I'm all right at home at the moment though. I wouldn't leave my mam.' She feels closer to her since her dad died. On the other hand, if her mam was able to look after herself, well, then she would move out with a clear conscience.

MARK SAMUELS

Mark Samuels is twenty years old. He lives in a three-bedroom, semi-detached council house with his wife, Tammy, and their baby son, Ryan, aged three months. They have a car but no telephone. Mark is presently on the dole, although he has worked. For over two years he was employed as a car mechanic before taking a job as a gravedigger and, later, working in the furnaces at a crematorium. 'Well I got sacked from mechanic's for fighting and the other one, it's a long story. . . . It just blitzed my head.' To date he has accumulated sixteen criminal convictions, mainly for offences to do with cars and violence. He has been sentenced to probation and community service and has served time in container units and prison. Tammy has two children from a previous relationship but both are in care.

Mark is of average height and about fifteen stones in weight. He has dark hair, cut short and brushed back at the sides. His moustache had grown into a beard by our second meeting. Wearing black jeans, black T-shirt, black boots and a rash of tattoos, he chain-smoked through the interviews. Although not overtly friendly, he talked freely and openly about himself and his family. He had agreed to take part, he said, 'because my mum asked me if I would'.

Mark is the oldest of five children. His two younger brothers, aged eighteen and thirteen, both of whom have learning difficulties, and his two sisters, aged sixteen and eleven, still live at home with their mother, who also has learning difficulties. Mark's parents divorced eleven years ago when his father went to live with another woman whom he later married. His father died recently from a heart attack at the age of forty-four. Mark has never liked his dad's second wife: 'We don't get on. . . . She never did nowt for him – he had to do everything his self – and she started fooling with other blokes behind his back.' After his father died his new wife brought Mark his watch: 'I wouldn't have took it if she'd have bought it. It's only because it was, like, my old feller's watch, that's why I took it.'

As a small child, Mark recalls living close to all his grandparents, although he remembers them as fairly elderly. All are now dead. When his first brother was born, Mark, whose father was often violent towards him, went to live with his mother's parents. 'He used to smack me around. It's like my dad didn't want me. He just pushed me out.' He stayed with his grandparents for a year, until his first sister was born, when he had to move back home because his grandfather developed angina. He remembers aunts and uncles being around, and he still maintains regular contact with his cousins.

Mark's parents had attended the same special school as children and had gone on to marry in their early twenties. His father used to have a job emptying dustbins although he was plagued by ill health, including asthma, angina, diabetes and three strokes, for much of his life. His mother too had worked until she married. It was she who had done most of the jobs around the house: his father had done next to nothing. The grandparents helped out at times, and his sister lent a hand with the washing up, shopping and cleaning as she grew older. Mark kept the gardens tidy.

Although he enjoyed his junior school, Mark was unhappy and never settled after he moved into the seniors. He found his teachers unsupportive, he was bored, and he truanted: 'Didn't like school, full stop.' Apart, that is, from school dinners when curries were his favourite: 'I'm like my old feller, sweet and sour.' Punishment was frequent and brutal. Teachers used a plimsoll, a ruler and a leather strap. Mark feels he received so much physical punishment that he became addicted to it: 'I used to like it, you know, the pain in my hands.' He stopped attending regularly at the age of thirteen. Finally he was expelled: 'I didn't want to do nowt, me. I just wanted to be shot of it.'

Even before he reached his teens he had been under a 'shrink' and was on medication 'for being a schizophrenic'. His mother had been unable to control him. He spent a year in a 'hospital type thing' when he was nine after smashing up his mum's house: 'It was for kids that were bad tempered, but they never calmed me down.' He recalls defending himself violently against taunts of being 'a child molester's son' when his father started going with his second wife who was only fifteen at the time: 'She were still at school and I got copped for it.' One lad who tormented him ended up in a coma after Mark repeatedly 'rammed his head into post of swings' and 'left him for dead'.

Mark feels he took on responsibility for the family when his father left home. He saw his duty as protecting his brothers and sisters from 'outsiders'. His mother used to be a member of the Salvation Army and twice they paid for the family to go on holiday. Mark, however, chose to stay at home and look after the house. He thinks one of the most important things his mother needed, and still does, is some form of respite, especially having two boys with learning difficulties:

> We used to have a social worker when my mum and dad split up. She were supposed to be helping but all she kept giving my mum were grief so I threw her through door. It's summat she said, and it got me into a bad mood. It got my mum upset . . . the kids, these lot, were crying. Told her if she ever got back in, she wouldn't get back out.

Mark was never short of friends to share his enthusiasm for push-bikes and skateboards and, later, motorbikes and cars. He was a member of the Boys Brigade, becoming an army cadet and then joining the Territorial Army. As a teenager he had been keen on kick-boxing, body building, weight training and power lifting, even winning some trophies. By the time he was fifteen, he had left home and was living with a girl-friend: 'I've been back on the odd times but I've always left, like, two week after.' He used to keep a python in a large tank in his mum's back room until she told him to get rid of it after it attacked her dog.

He began to get into trouble with the police from an early age, mainly for violence or offences related to cars. Over the years he has destroyed property and injured classmates, girlfriends, his mother and sister and many others: 'I've always battered them . . . my mum, she's frightened of me as well.' Mark hit his mother just the once. She had been trying to stop him beating his girlfriend.

> I mean, I don't know what's happening when I go into proper moods. I won't know what's happening, I won't even know what I've done. I can smash somebody and not even remember it, won't even know I've hit them.

He's used drugs (amphetamines and cannabis) but says, 'I like alcohol, I drink more than anything.' He refuses to take the medication he has been prescribed.

> I've always been black sheep of family anyway. I'm well known for, like, beating, violence, like that. First time I moved in here I caused trouble with him next door. I went for him with an axe. It's like my dad used to get in trouble with law. I've followed in his footsteps.

Mark feels he had a happy childhood: 'I had my freedom. I didn't have a care in the world. I was my own person.' He'd always had a close rela-tionship with his mother but not with his father who, he says, was an alcoholic like his grandfather. Even so, his father's death had been a shock. Mark feels some sadness because he'd been trying to get closer to his father of late: 'We got on since I've been the age I am now, up to his dying. Before he died, like, we started getting close.'

Mark has been unemployed for nineteen months and would like a job as a security guard:

> But nobody'll have me. Can't get on security because I've got a criminal record, and I've got tattoos. I went in for my City and Guilds doing motor mechanics. I passed everything apart from my electrics. I just do my own car now. I buy them, do them up, sell them . . . that's all I do, all day, now.

He still sees his mother most days and helps her with anything she needs doing: 'She's got me and my wife to help her out.' His oldest sister also spends a lot of time at his house and has made quite a few friends in the area. He makes sure she's in for half past ten though, 'I won't let her out any later.'

Mark knows where his loyalties lie.

> Well, we're a big family and if we need help I've always thought, like, there's me and our Dan – that's my cousin – we're both same age, we're both stocky lads, so if my mum gets trouble we're down here. My mum doesn't need anybody else to help her out while we're about.

His mother had recently called out the police twice when kids were throwing stones at her window:

> They never bothered, didn't even want to know, so I said, right, I'll deal with it in my own way. Copper says, 'You're going to get done for it then.' I says, if you sort him out, I says, I'll leave him alone.

Mark says he can only remember bits of his past: 'It's like since I got older, I just don't bother with my past.' But he recalls a few happy times:

> Like, I used to help my dad with cars, doing his car, and used to be driving out with him. I used to just spend most of my nights round at my grandparents. I was more close to my grandparents than what I was to my own parents . . . because of my old feller.

He often argued with his mum:

> Me and my mum didn't speak for months on end and then we started speaking, then we don't, then it's more arguing and I'll walk

out, get in the car and go home and I'll walk the street for the night and then I'll come back the next day.

The arguments are usually for the same reason: 'It's mainly because I'm always in trouble with police. She doesn't like me getting in trouble.'

Mark has now been married eleven months: 'I wanted to settle down because I were sick of getting in trouble with law.' Having a baby son has made him more aware. 'I know what I'd never do. I'd never hurt him. I'd hurt anybody who hurt him.' Summing up his character he says, 'I'm a passive person but I'm very violent with it. I've never thought about killing anybody. I like bruising them, like breaking a few bones, but never gone as far as killing anybody.'

At the last interview Mark was waiting for the vicar to call to make the final arrangements for his son's christening. The baby would be wearing the same christening robe that his dad had worn.

ADAM LLOYD

Thirty years old, over six feet tall, his dark hair cut short, Adam Lloyd sits in what had once been the front room of the two-bedroom council house he shares with his girlfriend and two of her children. The wall has been knocked through into the back parlour to make one large, and attractively furnished, living room. The house is situated on a small estate in the centre of a former mining village. The pit has now closed. The estate has recently been renovated and the houses have all had double-glazing and central heating installed. Adam, polite and quietly spoken, is dressed in jeans, sweatshirt and trainers. He launches straight into his story and talks easily for almost two hours, occasionally twiddling an earring.

Two years ago his partner left him taking their three children with her. 'I've got little lad and two little lasses.' Now he just sees them at weekends although they still live fairly close by. He also has two lurchers which he keeps for rabbiting.

Adam's mother had 'been taken advantage of' by a man for whom she used to babysit. Adam has never been told his father's name but believes he still lives locally. He had been a large baby, over eleven pounds at birth, and his mother had been put under some pressure by 'the Welfare' to have him adopted. His grandparents 'just hit roof'. They 'says, "No way. You're not adopting him. She's keeping him herself." They says, "We'll help her fetch him up as her own," and they did.' Three of his mother's brothers were living at home at the time and one, Robert, also had learning difficulties, like Adam's mother. Two of his uncles moved out while Adam was still a child but he remembers living in the family home with his mother, his grandparents and his Uncle Robert until he was twelve. Uncle Robert 'were one of these, when I were young, if I did owt wrong he wouldn't let them take it out on me. He used to stick up for me. He didn't like nobody hurting me.'

Adam's mother was an active woman and he recalls clearly how she 'used to go walking, and everywhere she went she used to take me – just to show me off, like – like they did in them days.'

Adam was a happy boy and spent a great deal of his time outside with his friends or uncles. His mother and grandparents, however, were very protective: 'They didn't like dark. Soon as it got dark, that were it. If I weren't in, used to come looking for me – my mother, our Robert, dog and all lot.' Even at eighteen they didn't like him going out at night. 'My mother and my grandma, they used to sit up worrying where I'd got to.' Adam's cousin finally had a word with them and told them to stop worrying and just give him his own key:

> And they started that, and they kept awake because sometimes I used to come in – they'd be in bed but they'd still be awake – and then she used to shout down, 'Who's that?'. I said, it's only me, like, and that were it then.

Adam didn't care much for school and often played truant. His one love was football. His granddad had turned out for the village team as a youth and he encouraged Adam as a small boy. Once bitten, Adam played every spare moment of the day, often not getting home for tea until after dusk. 'My mother says, "They used to have thy tea ready on table. Thy used to come in, take your school clothes off, put playing out clothes on," she says, "get your football boots, get football and straight out."' As a teenager, he once had a trial for Manchester City. A serious knee injury later cut short his playing days.

His grandfather used to work at the local pit, where he was in charge of the pit ponies, until he retired with a lung infection, and one of his lungs had to be removed. Adam's mother and grandma shared the housework. Adam slept in the same room as his mother, but it was always his granddad that soothed him to sleep whenever he was disturbed:

> He said, 'I'll get him to sleep,' my mother used to tell me. 'He used to go downstairs,' she says, 'sit in rocking chair, sing to you and in

five minutes you'd be gone.' She says, 'There were only him who could do it.'

Adam remembers having to take his punishment as a lad, but no more than any of his friends. 'They used to hit me with belt and that, my granddad. My mother used to hit me with her hand, but she would never hit me on head, just on my legs.'

Adam's grandfather died when he was twelve years old. He was devastated by the loss. His behaviour at home gradually became uncontrollable. and he refused to go to school. He admits, 'I started getting out of hand.' Eventually things reached a pitch where he was put into a children's home, and then another, and then an adolescent unit. For his mother and grandmother, he knows, having him taken away 'broke their heart, aye'. They used to visit him every weekend and ring every night at eight o'clock. Occasionally he would be allowed home and later he came for the long summer holidays. He began smoking but, knowing his family didn't approve, he always hid his cigarettes outside before going into the house. Twice he tried to escape, and walked the ten miles home: 'That's the first time we had police come.' The children's homes were no more successful at bringing him to heel than his mother and grandmother had been. At eighteen he was sent to an open prison.

The family had had a social worker from when Adam was a young child:

She was brilliant, all family could get on with her. Then she left to have a bairn and they give me another one, and she were a monster, her. I hated her. She was one of these who were right cocky. Like, 'You've got to do this,' 'Sit there,' 'Don't move'. I thought, well, if I can't get rid of you one way I'll get rid of you another. So I didn't used to talk to her.

His ruse worked and he was assigned a social worker he did like. 'Got me another one, a bloke, he were brilliant him. Because of him, I think that's how I got out of that prison in Leeds.'

Once I got into prison I settled down and I thought, well, my grandma's getting old, my mother's getting old with worry and that. . . . I thought, well, I'm going to get out before owt happens to them, and I just quietened down. I were in there six month, then I were out. And I thought, well, if I'd done that in first place I wouldn't have had to go in these different kids' homes, like. If I'd done that in first kids' home I went in, I'd have been out when I were sixteen, fifteen. When you get in these kids' homes, there's some in there who's in for robbery and all that, break-ins and that, and once you get mixed up with them it all goes funny then.

When he came home at nineteen he was determined to make up for lost time.

I did owt for her. I used to do shopping for them at weekends, mend fire, get coal in, and all lot. I blame myself . . . but they were a bit – my grandma, and my granddad and my mother – a bit too soft with me, like. Just more or less let me get my own road.

Adam has had a series of labouring jobs but is unemployed at present. His mother and Uncle Robert live in the family home just a few houses away. A nephew sleeps with them to make sure they're all right during the night. They both attend the local Adult Education Centre. Adam's mother, now a 51-year-old granny, began at the centre when she was sixteen and has been going ever since. His new girlfriend recalls seeing her around when she was a youngster: 'We used to call her names when we were at school. Well, I mean we were only eight year old, weren't we?'
Adam is still mindful of how other people see his mother:

These young uns live next door to my mother. We were in boozer, like, and she says, 'Oh, we've got two right idiots next door,' she says, 'both handicapped, they're both thick, like.' I just flipped when they'd said that about them. Same when I were at school, but I always used to put my fist first instead of my mouth, like. When I got older like, when they used to take mickey out of my mother and our Robert, I thought, well, instead of using my fist, use my mouth.

Adam's girlfriend avers, 'Bring his mother down, that's it, he goes crazy, don't you?'
He remembers his mother going to the 'Tec' at one time and bringing back some homework: 'She used to say, "Will thou do this for me?" I used to say, "No, I'll not do it for you. I'll help you." I says, "If I do it, you're not learning it."'
When his own children come over to stay at weekends, Adam says there's always one thing they want to do – go down the road and see their grandma. Like most grandparents, she spoils them. Adam's mother calls round most days to see him. She often babysits too when her grandchildren are staying with him. 'She's soft as a brush . . . and they knew she was. They knew that owt they asked for she'd give it 'em.' Adam also knows that she'll give him anything he asks for too: 'She's best mother I've had. They've got to give them a chance – haven't they?

– all these handicapped people. My mother got chance, and that were thirty year ago, and there's nowt wrong with me, like.'

VERONICA STEPHENSON

At a little over five feet tall, Veronica, with her short brown hair and ready smile, looks younger than her twenty-seven years. She is friendly, talkative and confiding. At present she is living in a hostel for young people with mental health problems on the outskirts of a former mill town in the heavy woollen district of the old West Riding of Yorkshire. She has a boyfriend quite a bit younger than herself and they are hoping to get engaged soon.

Veronica suffers from epilepsy, now controlled by medication. She takes an array of other tablets, mainly tranquillisers of one sort or another, and also has monthly injections 'to calm me down'. After these injections, her usual chatty self dissolves into unresponsiveness. In addition to the support she receives from her hostel staff, and from the 24-hour duty staff at a drop-in centre she uses, Veronica visits her GP regularly and is seeing a psychiatrist, a counsellor and an occupational therapist. She also belongs to a survivors' group. She finds most of these professionals helpful, except for the male psychiatrist who frustrates her when she tries to tell him how she feels. He dismisses her vulnerability and tells her that men act the way they do towards her because she gives them the wrong signals.

As a child, Veronica lived with her mother and father, and a brother who is just a year older. She has another brother, eight years older, but he was placed in a children's home as a baby. Her mother has learning difficulties, and Veronica has always thought of her as being 'ill'. Her father too, who has a painful disability in his legs, missed out on most of his schooling. Neither of them can read or write. Her parents separated recently although the family, excepting the oldest brother, remain in close contact with one another. Veronica was one of the people in the study who agreed to write her own story. This is what she penned:

> As a young girl me and my brother Conrad lived with our parents at Winthrop Moor my mum was ill so it meant that Dad made our meals and took us to School and brought us own from School.
>
> Dad had to make sure that we were in bed before he went to work at night as my mum coudent see to us as my dad worked nights on a twelve hour shift.
>
> So that meant he was not getting much sleep as he had to be

there for us when we went to school and to be there for us when we came home from school so he new we would be alright before he went to work.

As we got older me and my brother relised that Mum couldent do much for us. So we helped around the house helping mum and dad as much as we could.

We then moved to Helmsall where we both made a lot of friends we went to school with them and played out until it was time to come in for a bath or go to bed.

Our parents also took us on holiday and day trips we had lots of fun enjoyed our self as a family and we went out to different places every day so we didnt stop in the same place.

Social worker would also come round to the house to see how mum and dad was coping with us and to see if they needed any help with any thing.

When I was six years old I can remember going to this family for a week away from my parents and brother.

There was this girl she was a year younger than me I had a great time while I was they took me out and I played hours with this girl but I never understood why I went away from my parents and brother. the social worker never told me they just said that I was going away for a little holiday. When I was 9 and Conrad was 10 we was taken off our parents we was taken into a childrens home we were taken in to Moorfield Park at Winthrop The reason why we went in there was because the social worker was acusing my dad of hitting me and my brother.

So they took us under care for twenty eight days after them 28 days the social services took it to court so that meant we had to stay in the childrens home untill we was 15 or 16 years old.

Every six months it kept going back to court to see if my parents could get the care order dropped so that they could take us both home.

But the social services always won the case they made me feel very angry with not letting Conrad and I go home for good at that age we couldent understand why they were doing this.

After Conrad had been at Moorfield Park for three years he decided that that home wasent for him that the other children was a lot younger than he was so they moved him to Scardale where there was boys his own age he could go around with and to make friends.

Conrad came out of the home when he was 16 years old and I went home for good when I was 15 years old as soon as I came home

I took the social services to court and got the care order taken off me. I was glad to be free of them I didn't like them they did a lot of harm to our family.

When I was 13 my eldest brother Tony abused me he was touching me down below and he tried to have sex with me that made me destructive at School I was allways throwing tables and chairs about and fighting because the other kids was picking on me as I was to quiet and they thought that there was something wrong with me.

The head at the School was going to send me to a Special School they thought that there was something wrong with me.

At 15½ years old my dad started to have sex with me that happend every time we was alone which was quite a lot as Mum was out shopping or at Friends and Conrad was too out with his friends. This went on for six months Dad also used to call me his misstress and not to tell anbody what he had been doings he said that nobody would belive me. After that I have been raped sexualy abused by people who I know and people I dont know. This as carried on untill I have reached 27 years of age.

I have taken them to the police but there wasent enough eveidence for it to go to court but when I was raped I got £5000 compensation but that dosent ease the pain I have to go through all my life Thinking about what hurt people have done to me.

I have taken overdoses tried to cut my arms and wrists I just wanted to die not to rember what had happed I wanted total piece.

I saw a counsellor who helped me a lot I saw her for two and ½ years I missed her when I couldent see her any more as I got on very well with her I could tell her anything about me. Then she left to go in to another job and that meant I couldent see her any more that made me sad as I could tell her any thing about me. and she would do what she could to help me.

In September of last year I got two new key workers at Heathcroft house in Darford.

There names are Deidre Angler and Josie Baker. They come to see me when they can but I go to see them at Heathcroft house.

Heathcroft house is a place where I can go for company they have a drop in service which means that people like me can go to the drop in for 9 in the morning to 9 at night.

I have also been on respite there for two seprate weeks. as I have been having a crisis and couldent cope on my own. so I was took in there for a rest. They also have a twenty four hour phone line so I can phone any time of the day or night if I need to talk to any body.

I am now living at Edge End Hostel in Winthrop I live with five other people.

and there is staff from monday to saturday. After I have been there a short while I will get my own place and try and settle down and to live my life.

Veronica's bedroom is full of soft toys she has collected or been given over the years, and a number of photos. These photos are mainly of babies and children belonging to her brothers and friends. She would like to become a nanny or at least work with children. She'd also like a baby of her own: 'I'd give it a lot of love . . . and I'd give it a lot of cuddles.' She says her own mother 'never used to cuddle me or hold me or anything like that. My dad doesn't either. I think I missed that as a child.'

She says she doesn't see her parents as much now, but she still visits her mother at least four times a week:

I still go up and see her, still love her, but I can't talk to her. She doesn't understand me when I talk to her. She doesn't want to listen to me. She tells me what's gone on through the day and that.

A little while after a letter, headed Edge End Hostel, arrived:

I am still feeling down and am harming my self I have told the staff what I am doing to my self and they said when I feel like that I have to talk to someone.

I am sick of feeling like this I wish that I could turn the clocks back so none of this would have happend.

I sometimes wish that I wasent hear. when I have taken overdoses I wish that I had died

Then I wouldent have to relive all this pain.

Love from Veronica XXX

BOXING LIVES

The problem of arriving at any sort of overall appraisal of the significance of having been brought up by parents with learning difficulties is underscored by the complexity of people's lives and the many different ways of interpreting their experience. Several practical issues have to be addressed in trying to assess how well people have managed the transition to adulthood:

Whose standards?

A key question, as Edgerton and Bercovici (1976) point out, is whose criteria of success to use, 'ours or theirs'. Do we as researchers impose our own external standards of adjustment or do we adopt the standards that people use in their own lives? This choice is given added weight by the fact that personal happiness and satisfaction with one's lot are not directly related to positive adaptation in life (Werner, 1989). Judged by the values of the wider society, Mark Samuels might appear a pretty wild character whose appetite for violence suggests some deep-seated disturbance. For his own part, Mark is unapologetic for his thuggery, seeing it as within the limits of the tough community in which he lives and necessary at times to protect his family.

Opportunities and expectations

Are the same criteria to be used for people with and people without learning difficulties? Most people with learning difficulties never attain the trappings of adult status: a job, a wage, a driver's licence, credit cards, a mortgage, a home of their own, marriage, children and the like. These are the outward markers of independence and responsibility that constitute the social meaning of adulthood. They define a threshold beyond which few men and women with learning difficulties pass: a fact which contributes to the deep-rooted cultural perception of them as perennial children. This image or stereotype in turn feeds back to shape their own identity and sense of self.

Against this background of social exclusion and repression, it could be misleading to look at what people have made of their lives through the same lens as used for those who have not encountered the same disadvantages. Bonnie Craven has achieved few of the things that most people in their thirties would take for granted. She is still living at home with her mum, she has few friends, little social life, no qualifications, no job, no income of her own and no boyfriend. On the other hand, she lives in an ordinary neighbourhood where she has deep roots and encounters no harassment, she enjoys a stable and secure family life, is mainly responsible for the running of the household, looks after her mother and sister, and shows a happy face to the world. In these ways, she has a measure of control over her own life and a presence in the community not shared by the majority of people with learning difficulties. Any attempt to explore how people's lives have turned out must at some point make allowance for the different expectations and opportunities extended to the likes of Bonnie Craven.

Parenting in context

Parenting is not usually a task undertaken by parents alone. Mothers and fathers are often not the only people involved in bringing up children. Other people may contribute, including members of the extended family, older brothers and sisters, friends and neighbours, and professional helpers. The quality of parenting a child receives depends not only on the skills and competence of his or her parents but also on the strength of this wider network and the availability of other parent-figures. Adequate supports can compensate for shortcomings in the skills of parents to ensure satisfactory care for the child. Whereas being a parent defines a biological relationship, the process of parenting constitutes a set of social relationships which is variable and negotiable. Whereas Adam Lloyd spent the early years of his life in a household made up of his maternal grandparents, his mother and three uncles (until two moved out leaving just his Uncle Robert), Veronica Stephenson's mum and dad had lost all contact with their relatives, including their own parents, and looked after her and her brother without any outside support until the social services intervened to break up the family. These examples underline the importance of looking at parenting in context, at the shared or collective aspects of parenting and not just the competence of parents, when trying to interpret the links between child-rearing, children's development and adaptation in later life.

Confounding factors

A fundamental problem in trying to unravel the later life effects of having been brought up by a mother and/or father with learning difficulties is separating the outcomes attributable to parenting from those resulting from other confounding factors, most especially poverty and deprivation. Parents with learning difficulties are generally relegated to living in conditions and under pressures that foster child care problems and make it hard for anyone to be a good parent (Gath, 1988; Rosenburg and McTate, 1982; Schilling et al., 1982; Unger and Howes, 1986). Many of the adults in this study had experienced an emotionally thorny childhood in which broken homes, victimisation, physical abuse and sexual molestation figured prominently. Differentiating the impact of such traumas from the effects of having a parent or parents with learning difficulties is a puzzle.

Veronica Stephenson's story illustrates the point. It is not easy to unpick the relative contribution that family pathology, separation from parents and admission into care, and sexual exploitation have made to her vulnerability, low self-esteem and suicidal impulses. The danger is of simply putting all her troubles down to having a mother with learning difficulties.

The classic research solution to this type of problem is to use a comparison group of parents without learning difficulties to control for factors other than the variable under study. This design was not a practical option in this case for reasons rehearsed by Stoneman (1989). It was not possible to pinpoint in advance the factors for which it was necessary to control and the range is almost certainly too great to make close matching possible. For example, given the importance of relatives and other benefactors in supporting mothers and fathers with learning difficulties, a proper comparison study would involve matching across the parents' wider family and social network. Equally, it would entail controlling for the input from professionals and the services given their key role in supporting or undermining parental competence (Booth and Booth, 1993; Tucker and Johnson, 1989). Practical difficulties of identification, recruitment and retention make these objectives unrealistic yet, as Stoneman comments, without such careful matching 'comparison groups can be potentially harmful'.

Life-cycle effects

The job of reaching a view about how successfully people have come through their own childhood and established themselves in the adult world is made harder by the fact that lives move on whereas a study such as this provides only a snapshot in time. The implication of this simple point is that the outcomes being measured can never be regarded as fixed or final. Werner (1989), for example, followed a large cohort of high-risk children from the prenatal period into adulthood and found the effects of a stressful childhood varied at different stages of the life cycle as the balance between risk and protective factors in people's lives changed.

This can be seen in the stories recounted above. Adam Lloyd admits to getting out of hand in his youth but settled down with the help of his social worker after a short spell in prison. Mark Samuels reckons he got married in the hope that the extra responsibility might calm him down and keep him out of trouble. The lesson here is that any summary judgement of people's adaptive functioning is influenced by the point at which one enters their lives.

At the time we met her, Veronica Stephenson was not sure life was worth the living. Yet we might have found a very different person had we come across her later having, say, found new feelings of self-worth through the love of her boyfriend. Given that the people in this study included some just leaving adolescence and some entering middle age, the likelihood is that their stories will be marked by such 'life-cycle effects'.

Meaningful lives

Trying to understand how people's lives have been influenced by having a parent with learning difficulties involves knowing something about what they make of their own past. This goes beyond merely establishing the bald facts of people's experience to get at the significance they attach to them. Formal methods of measurement are not capable of handling the inconsistencies, contradictions, idiosyncrasies and complexities that characterise this sort of interpretive data. Lives are not easily squeezed into boxes. The strength of narrative methods, on the other hand, is precisely that they provide a way of accessing lives at the level of lived experience which allows the incorporation of feeling into knowing. On the downside, however, their use entails the loss of the capacity for aggregation and statistical generalisation.

Scheherazade's dictum

We have not resolved these research dilemmas, although for better or worse we have decided how to deal with them in this study. Our aim is to treat the individual as a microcosm (following Scheherazade's dictum that 'one life is simply all lives lived separately') as a means of making the personal general. Our analysis will be bounded by the stories we have been told. One problem with this narrative approach is that the stories generated tend to be long on words and their insights are not easily summarised, unlike data that can be reduced to numbers, compressed into tables and projected on overheads. For this reason, the rest of this chapter will attempt to step back a little from the details and particulars of individual lives in order to provide a comparative assessment of how the adult children in our study have come through what would generally be seen as a risk-filled upbringing by parents with learning difficulties.

DIMENSIONS OF WELL-BEING

The accounts of lives provided by the people in our study were used to develop a range of indicators for gauging personal outcomes across a number of dimensions of living based on their own reported experience, supplemented where appropriate by observational material. In this section, we show how each one of these indicators was defined, present the data, highlight any problems of interpretation and offer a brief commentary on the findings.

Physical growth and health

Information about people's health status was collected by observation and questioning. We had no access to medical records and no clinical assessment was undertaken. In this respect, our data must be treated with the same reservations as apply to most general health surveys that rely on self-report as a basis for assessment. An overall health index was compiled from each individual's personal history taking into account the following facts gathered from the interviews: above-average weight, under-average height, mainly poor health as a child, evidence of mental health problems at some time, a disability or other long-term medical problem, lengthy periods in hospital, attempted suicide.

Seven people presented none of these risk factors; no-one showed them all. The most frequently recorded problem (twelve cases) was being overweight (which affected all seven women with learning difficulties). Half (six) of this group exhibited none of the other indicators. Eleven people reported having a disability (other than learning difficulties) or a long-term health problem, the most common falling into a category including asthma, epilepsy, speech impairment and dyslexia. Seven people had experienced mental health problems, of whom two had attempted suicide. No-one exceeded a tally of four risk factors, but psychiatric troubles were implicated in three of the four cases with the poorest health rating in the study. Just three people said they had mainly poor health as a child.

The now-adult children in the study divide into four broad groups on the basis of their health status:

- People with learning difficulties mostly in good health except for some, especially the women, being overweight.
- People without learning difficulties but with a history of mental health problems and associated troubles.
- People without learning difficulties having a mainly clear health record.
- A small number of people from each of the above categories with some form of chronic illness or impairment.

It is not easy to draw any conclusions from this breakdown. There are undoubtedly more people with learning difficulties than would be expected in a similar group drawn randomly from the general population. However, as explained in chapter 2, it is not possible to say whether this is due to the effects of genetic inheritance, a deprived upbringing, institutional discrimination or whether it is an artefact of the study. Equally, there are more people with mental health problems than would be found in a cross-section of the population at large but, again, it is important to be wary of making too hasty a connection between this fact and the quality of parenting people received. Individual stories show that other factors were certainly implicated in people's psychiatric troubles, including having children taken away, sexual abuse (always by someone other than the parent(s) with learning difficulties) and system abuse (see chapter 9).

Friends and peer relationships

People were sorted according to their 'mateyness' as children using their own accounts of friendships and play routines to identify those who had a mostly lonely, isolated childhood, through those with few but some friends, to those who were relatively gregarious. Specific information used to classify individuals in this way included the number of friends mentioned, the range of activities they shared together, and whether they visited each other's houses, played in the street or saw each other only at school.

Eight people spoke of a childhood spent without friends or regular playmates, largely cut off from other kids at home and at school. By contrast, nine people gave accounts picturing a childhood full of friends. The remainder fell into the middling category or shifted from one to another as they grew older. There were no apparent gender differences in patterns of friendship. Martin Riddick and Andy Ambler illustrate these extremes in personal terms:

Martin Riddick

Martin has always had close friends. As a child in mainstream school he would spend a great deal of time with them, going to the pictures, and to the Saturday football, playing round their houses and later going to the pub. When he decided to move right away from his family to find work, even then he went with some of his friends. 'I've always been able to make friends very easy.' On returning to live in his home town many years later, he found his old friends were few on the ground: 'It were a case of making friends all over again really, night school, getting involved in squash and badminton, getting involved in different activities.'

Andy Ambler

Andy was an only child and quite a lonely little boy. Living in a house of adults, he only saw other children at the special school to which he was bussed every day. The other children in the neighbourhood who were his age attended the local school and he didn't play with them. He only remembers one friend ever coming round his house. His mum had always taught him, 'not to mix with the wrong people'. He did have two girlfriends when he was thirteen but these relationships were short-lived. Only when he got to fifteen did he sometimes go out on a Sunday and play football with some local lads. He suffered a great deal from other kids 'tormenting me for no reason'. Looking back he feels his mother over-protected him.

Such variations in experience, mirrored in the study group as a whole, suggest that limited friendship networks in childhood cannot be explained simply in terms of parental characteristics or parenting behaviour. All but one of the most socially isolated children had learning difficulties. Over and above the sort of parental over-protectiveness of which Andy Ambler speaks, children with learning difficulties are also segregated from their peers by processes of social exclusion within local communities and the educational system. Family composition and changes in the make-up of the family also have a bearing on children's friendships. Lone children were more likely to have fewer friends. The separation of parents or being taken into care broke up friendships and sometimes made it hard for children to form new relationships. Finally, changing schools, and especially moving from junior to secondary school, also reshaped children's networks for better or worse. Against this background, if the experience of the people in our study is anything to go by, sociability in childhood is as likely to be affected by factors outside as inside the home, and certainly should not be seen through the window of the parents' learning difficulties alone.

Functioning in the school environment

How did the now-adult children in our study get on at school and college? On the outcomes side, their educational careers were appraised in terms of progress and attainment and, on the process side, in terms of problems and sanctions.

Attainment was assessed using the following indicators: qualifications obtained; evidence of ability at sports; progression to further or higher education. Problems were defined as including: being suspended; absenteeism and truancy; frequent punishment; being bullied; and having few school friends.

Problems were more in evidence than achievements at school. Only four people left with any qualifications; none had gone into higher education. Sixteen people, of whom ten had learning difficulties, had either been to or were attending a further education college. By contrast, four people had been suspended from school, fifteen experienced persistent bullying, and thirteen (of whom only three had learning difficulties) confessed to regularly skipping school. Although people with learning difficulties notched up fewer achievements at school – and noticeably reported having fewer school friends – they also ranked lower in terms of problem behaviours. Keith Riddick, Callum Johnson and Amy Norris illustrate the contrasting experiences within the group.

Keith Riddick

Keith enjoyed his schooldays and made many friends. A neighbour's son was his best friend throughout his school career and he has always remained in close contact with him. Keith played football for the school and left at sixteen with GCE 'O' levels in English, maths and history, and six CSEs. Although he didn't continue his education at that stage, today he is seriously thinking of enrolling at college to do a computer course.

Callum Johnson

Callum attended both special and mainstream schools but liked neither. School, he says, 'was like a prison'. His mum always had problems getting him up on Monday mornings because, 'I didn't like going.' He didn't enjoy schoolwork, finding the writing hard. Cooking, he says, especially baking cakes, was 'the best work I liked to do at school'. He didn't like his teachers who 'used to tell me off and that, and I'd swear at them. They kept putting me against the wall and all that when I did something wrong.' He remembers the telling-off he used to get from the headmaster for swearing at staff and sometimes hitting other children. Although he thought the other kids at school were mostly 'all right', he admits that he got bullied and called names he didn't like, such as 'spaz' and 'idiot'. He left at sixteen and now attends an Adult Training Centre where, he feels, they treat him better than at school: 'It's all right down here. You get more attention down here. They asked me about college but I said no. I don't want college.'

Amy Norris

Amy started truanting when she moved to secondary school at thirteen. She couldn't tolerate the bullying. A gang of girls 'took me up at St Mark's Church, round there, and kicked me. They just kicked me. That were every day for three weeks.' She told her teachers 'but they didn't do nowt'. Her auntie 'said that I could have dinner there and come down any time I want'. Soon she was only going to school one day a week and spending the rest of the time at her auntie's. Her mum and dad 'didn't find out'. She admits, 'I didn't learn owt at school.' Eventually she was sent to an adolescent unit where she spent twelve months on a residential basis and another year as a day attender while living at home. 'I did some exams at adolescent unit and I passed. I don't know what. I didn't even know I took some.' Asked what she liked most about her childhood Amy replied, 'Staying off school.' She is now attending a youth training centre.

There is a wide gulf between the educational careers and experience of the people with and without learning difficulties in our study group. There were very few like Keith Riddick who established close friendships at school, excelled at sport, kept out of trouble, passed his exams and is now thinking about going back to college. For the most part, the men and women without learning difficulties showed more similarities with Amy Norris' story of chronic under-achievement, persistent absenteeism or truanting, problems of learning, clashes with teachers, general disaffection with school life, and early leaving followed by unemployment.

The people with learning difficulties, on the other hand, presented a picture of their schooldays that does not differ in any marked respects from most of their peers. All attended special schools at some time and most (ten) had received all their education up to the age of sixteen in such settings. Their schooling passed with few problems of discipline, behaviour (although bullying and being bullied were no less common) or attendance, with few lasting friendships, and almost nothing in the way of formal achievements. However, fully two-thirds had moved on into continuing education and were attending courses at further education colleges, probably largely as a result of new opportunities introduced by the 1988 Education Reform Act. This contrasts with the 1989 Social Services Inspectorate finding that four out of five students at social services day centres had no experience of further education (Department of Health, 1989).

Overall, then, while the upbringing and family circumstances of the now-adult children without learning difficulties certainly did not make for their easy or successful passage through school, equally it did not in any way appear to jeopardise the school career of those with learning difficulties.

Family roles and relationships

An attempt was made to capture something of the subjective quality of family bonds for the now-adult children in the study using their own accounts of their feelings towards family members and, where relevant, their experiences of separation and relationships after leaving home.

Positive experiences of family life were held to be reflected in comments suggesting that a person felt himself or herself to have been a favoured member of the family; in positive expressions of feeling regarding parents, grandparents, siblings and other relatives; where people had maintained close contact with their parents or family after leaving home; and where contact with the family had been renewed after a period in care. Negative experiences were held to be indicated by the opposite of these feelings, and by having lost contact or having only limited contact with parents since leaving home.

Presenting this data is not easy. People's feelings and experiences did not fall unambiguously into one or the other category: many had both positive and negative things to say about their parents; some felt differently towards their mother than they did towards their father, or towards different brothers and sisters or different relatives; and, of course, people's feelings changed over time. Biographical reflections always provide a view of the past from a standpoint in the present and it is to be expected that people's relationships within their family will mirror something of their own position in the life cycle. Conrad Stephenson's story illustrates the point and shows how hard it is to freeze the ups and downs of everyday family relationships in a static coding frame:

Conrad Stephenson

Conrad, his wife Sally and their baby daughter, now nineteen months old, live in their own three-bedroom terrace house which they share with Sally's mum, who moved in shortly after their marriage when her husband died, and two large dogs.

As a young child, Conrad had lived with his mother and father and his younger sister. He has a half-brother, Tony, his mother's first-born, who is seven years his senior, but Tony was placed in a children's home as a baby and Conrad 'never saw him much until I got into sort of my teenage life'. Tony had returned home when he was sixteen but within a month or two he'd had a blazing row with his mother about money and 'my dad told him to leave us then. My parents don't get on with my older brother.' Since then Conrad has had only fleeting contact with him. A year or two back Tony had broken into Conrad's previous house and stolen some money. The family are now pledged to keep his new address and telephone number a secret from Tony.

Conrad was aware of having aunties and uncles as a child but 'with my mum's condition, nobody bothered with my mum, so it was very rare we went round to relatives or they came round to see us'. His dad was raised by his mother and three sisters and Conrad thinks they resented him getting married 'because they didn't like my mum'. His mother's own brothers and sisters 'never bothered with her either'. So apart from occasional visits to grandparents they had very little to do with the rest of the family.

Conrad looks back on his early childhood with happy memories:

I can remember, sort of when I was six, seven, eight, every summer, all the local children used to come into the back garden and we used to build like a Grand National out of tin cans to jump over and run round. We used to have little competitions and see who could get round this course the fastest. It was a big back garden and everybody used to come round in summer. I can remember one bonfire night we'd made a right big bonfire in the back garden. Everybody came round and because we lived in these sort of painted tin prefabs – we used to call it the bean can village – it blackened all the windows and all the paint blistered and started peeling off the outside. My dad got in a bit of trouble over it.

Up until he was ten the family went everywhere and did everything together. His dad was always the disciplinarian. Misbehaviour resulted in being sent to bed early: 'You'd have to march up the steps.' His mother never used to say anything. 'My dad used to do all the talking to us. My mum was a background figure. She was just there.' There was little physical affection from his parents – 'We didn't hug or anything' – but in other ways they were a close family.

When he was ten, Conrad and his sister were put in a children's home. Social services 'said we were going away for a month while my mum and dad had a rest'. Conrad feels the social worker should have realised sooner that his parents were having difficulties by the number of times the family trooped down to the local office: 'By the time they really investigated it was too late. To us they were just normal. To other people I think they would have been stressed, near to nervous breakdowns.' It was the first time he and his sister had been split up: 'I was at one end of the corridor and my sister was at the other end, so I could hear her crying, she could hear me crying.' After a month, 'I said, "Are we going home now?", and they says, "Oh no, you've got to go to court."'

Conrad and his sister remained in care for the next six years. It was then they learned to appreciate how much their parents cared for them: 'I think it showed the way they came to see us every week. Never missed. Even if there was six foot of snow they'd come.' He and Veronica 'used to stick like glue to each other, and wrestle, just to be together more or less' until finally they were split up and he was transferred to another children's home. The strong protective need to look after his sister that he felt during these years remains to this day.

After two years in the children's home, he started going home for a day, gradually lengthening into a weekend. As he got older he would sometimes pop in to see his mum and dad after school. At sixteen he went home for good, but things didn't work out: 'I think becoming a teenager, and my mum and dad still thinking I was nine or ten, I wanted to do things I wanted to do and they couldn't grasp that.' He moved out into his own flat.

One day he went to visit his mum and found her crying in a chair. 'What's wrong?', he asked her, and she told him his dad wanted a divorce. 'I says he can't do that, I'll go see him.' Conrad tracked him down at the local club. 'Look,' he said, 'you can't just throw thirty-odd years away. You've struggled this long you might as well carry on. Can't get any worse.' His dad told him it was nothing to do with him or his sister: 'Keep out of it.' Conrad 'chucked a pot of beer over his head and ran to his house and set it on fire and ran away.' Then he called the fire brigade. 'I was just getting my anger out.' He was sent to prison for eight months.

When he came out of prison, 'things started falling into place'. He and his father 'both had a good chat and said we were both wrong what we did. We resolved the differences and since then, you know, all my dad has to do is pick up phone and I'll be there really.' He is also the one his mum always turns to: 'I know my mum adores me, probably same way as I feel about her. I think she respects me as well, my mum, for what I've done.' Conrad recognises that his feelings towards his parents have changed. 'I think once you get older you start respecting them for what they are and what they've done, you know.' He sees himself as 'generally a bit soft' with his own daughter. 'I'm always hugging her. I think that's where it's different from my parents.'

Conrad's story adds a personal slant to most of the common features that ran through people's accounts of their family relationships:

- All but three (twenty-seven) people expressed positive feelings (of love, affection, gratitude, respect or the like) towards at least one of their parents, and in only three cases did these remarks specifically not refer to the parent with learning difficulties.
- Twenty-five people (including all the men) said they were close to their mother, and in twenty-two of these cases the mother had learning difficulties. Fewer people (eleven) expressed similar feelings about their father: twelve admitted to having a distant relationship with him and most of the rest had either never known him or had had no contact with him at all as a child.
- Every person in the study had maintained close contact with at least one of their parents (for so long as they were alive). This fact needs to be seen in the context of the study. Many people were located and contacted through their parent(s). Even so, the process of tracing potential respondents yielded very few parents who had lost contact with their child(ren) and the evidence seems to point to the enduring nature of parent-child bonds in these families.
- Every person who had spent time in care as a child had subsequently re-established contact with their surviving parent(s). There was no suggestion of people wanting to make a clean break with their past in order to establish an identity free from the stigma of having a parent with learning difficulties.
- A substantial majority of now-adult children without learning difficulties talked positively of their relationships with grandparents, at

least one sibling (although almost as many were critical of another), and other relatives. By contrast, fewer than half of those with learning difficulties expressed similar sentiments. No-one had anything bad to say about their grandparents.

* Two out of three people (twenty-one) passed some negative comments about their mother and/or father, although only a minority of people (eleven) spoke critically of a parent with learning difficulties. Ten people directed their grievances specifically at a father without learning difficulties.

The picture presented here challenges many prejudicial assumptions about the durability of relationships between children and parents with learning difficulties. People too often find it difficult to respect the authenticity of the feelings that underpin the bond between parent and child (Booth and Booth, 1994b). The fact remains, however, that the majority of people in this study had maintained a valued relationship with their families, often despite the threats to family continuity posed by the separation, divorce or death of their parents or their own reception into care. Most people remained close to the parent with learning difficulties (perhaps because this was usually the mother) even when families split up. Equally, most retained fond memories of a parent they had lost. It is hard to imagine that these responses would have been significantly different in the case of people without a parent who has learning difficulties. The general conclusion seems to be the obvious one: people love their parents despite and not because of who they are.

Memories of childhood

A small minority of people (three) looked back on their childhood with a blanket sense of unhappiness. Tina Wimpenny was one of them:

Tina Wimpenny

Tina's family lived next door to her grandmother and, as a child, Tina used to sleep in her granny's spare bedroom because there wasn't enough room for her at home. Money was always tight. She recalls her mother scratching to pay the rent and can't ever remember having any toys. Once, when she was about eleven, her father threw her downstairs causing grave internal injuries which have prevented her from having any children of her own. After this incident she was placed in a residential school where she never made any friends. Thinking back Tina says, 'I were sad all the time.' She still cries at the thought. She can't bring to mind anything from her younger days that had made her happy.

The great majority of people (twenty-one), however, said that they were mostly happy at home. Such comments usually found their resonance in accounts of lives marked by routine ordinariness in which happiness emerges as an absence of sadness or regrets rather than as remembered pleasures.

Life tended to deliver more knocks as people grew up so that more reported being happy as a young child than as a teenager. Eight people, like Conrad Stephenson above, said they had been happy up to being taken into care. Others recalled a happy home but had their lives made miserable by bullying at school or victimisation in the local community. For most people, the causes of whatever upsets darkened their memories of childhood originated either outside the home or from traumas like the death of a parent or close relative, or the break-up of their parents marriage. Betty Roberts is a case in point:

Betty Roberts

Betty's parents split up after a bitter argument when she was seventeen. Her father has learning difficulties and he went back to live with his own parents. As a little girl, Betty used to help him in the garden, and the family always used to do the shopping together. She liked her school and her teachers and had many friends there. The family all belonged to the RSPB and attended meetings of the local society regularly. Her mum and dad always made sure the three of them went together on any field trips. She also recalls many jolly family holidays by the sea. She has not seen her dad since he and her mum separated.

In the main, most people felt their family life as a child had been generally happy. Some acknowledged they sometimes had to go without 'if we hadn't got the money to buy stuff' but, significantly, only one person expressed regrets about not having 'parents like other families'. Most people made a distinction between 'going without' and 'missing out on' things. Shortage of money and chronic debt might have meant going without 'good clothes and that' or settling for 'whatever snap we could afford' but such deprivations did not necessarily lead people into thinking they were being short-changed. Asked whether he ever felt he was missing out on anything as a child, Conrad Stevenson spoke for others when he replied:

No, because that was the way of life, wasn't it? So, you know, I didn't bother what other people had. I got this and, OK, everybody else got their fancy gadgets what had come on the market. I got a cowboy outfit and a little action man and they'd got the latest sort of computer game that come out at the time. I wasn't bothered.

The experience of abuse

Sixteen people reported having experienced some form of physical and/or sexual abuse as a child, nine of whom had learning difficulties. In just over half of these cases (nine) the perpetrator was said to have been the victim's father. These accusations against fathers were mostly of physical abuse: just one daughter said she had been sexually molested. No mothers were cited for abuse. Abuse by parents with learning difficulties was rare: just one father was accused by his two now-adult children of having been physically violent to them.

Dennis Sutherland

Dennis lives with his parents, a younger brother and two younger sisters. He has inherited cataracts and has lost his sight in one eye. He has a volatile relationship with his father, who has learning difficulties: 'I don't get on with my dad.' His father was very violent towards all his children. 'He used to belt us with belt, hit us with fist, in face, anywhere he can get. One time he used to hit us on head.' Occasionally he would hit Dennis's mum too but she was not averse to hitting him back. Dennis says his father has now stopped hitting him though he still beats Dennis's youngest sister.

Eleven people said they had suffered physical (eight) and/or sexual (six) abuse at the hands of people other than or as well as their own father. There was no evidence to suggest that children with learning difficulties had been more vulnerable to exploitation from people outside the home. All the cases of physical abuse and one instance of sexual abuse involved a stepfather or stepmother:

Sonja Fenton

As a child, Sonja lived with her mother, stepfather and four brothers. She was the youngest in the family and never knew her real father. When she was twelve her mother died of cancer. Sonja continued living with her stepfather. He began to abuse her physically and sexually: 'Hit me with cane, hit me with frying pan in my face.' During the following years, she had two children by him: both babies were taken away at birth against her wishes. When her stepfather remarried, his new wife placed Sonja in a hostel.

Almost double the number of women (ten) as against men (six) had suffered some form of abuse: six from sexual abuse compared to none of the men. Four women had been victims of rape or incest as a child. Amy Norris was one of the people who agreed to write a short biographical sketch for us. She was keen to do it instead of the repetitive keyboard exercises that otherwise occupied most of her day on the youth training scheme she attended. Her neatly typed script, with few spelling mistakes but no punctuation, arrived through the post. It was probably the longest piece of continuous prose Amy had ever written:

MY LIFE

I was born the 14th april 1977 i lived up at the whitton on BASH-STREET ROAD we lived there for five years then we moved onto ivy close we lived on ivy wood crescent i went to montfort school we lived there four two years then we moved onto spitfire avenue i went to wellhouse nursery first school i was bullied there by some boys then eddie came down to my house for a couple of days there was me and eddie and brian and cilla in the bunk bed me eddie and brian was on top bed while james cilla on the bottom bed connie and james was in my mum and dads bed while my mum and dad was in the spare room then the first ever day we got a dog was lassy was from highwood kennels she was all white all over her body then my uncle said he would like her to live with us because they just moved from germany to england to live down here. two weeks before my nineth birthday i met charlie low then it cam two days before my nineth birthday i was rushing to get some clothes ready for the next day before my birthday came it was my mum's and my auntie's birthdaythey were 29 years old then i went with a friend of mine to town to meet charlie out side the kings head hewas there on time i told him what time i had to be back before nine' oclock i went with him to his flat he asked me to make some beans on toast for tea i made them and told them there tea was ready the came into the kitchen and ate all there tea charlie wanted to talk to denise because charlie took me down to the park to play on the swings then charlie

said it was time to go home so i ran up the stairs to the flat then i fell
asleep on the sette i heard charlie say leave her here for the night so
denise slept as well i was carried into the bed room half way through
the night i felt some body on top of me i woke up andsaid what are
you doing then i said dont you dare so he carried on then the next
morning i was ready to go home i just stept out side the door then i
saw the police riat van out side i went and told denise she said come
on then lets take you home now then the police came up stairs and
said are you amy norris i said yeas i am amy he said come on darling
lets take you down to the van i said what have i done wrong they said
no you have,nt done any thing wrong they bowt charlie out of the
flat and down to the van i got in the van and they took me home i
got into the house my uncle jim from germany was there then i got
changed my cousins came around and my friends joe burden mick
came around because they heard what had happened then this
police surgean came around and had a look at me they said i was
defenitally raped my friends heard what she said and came in and
said areyou alright amy isaid yes.

While the frequency of abuse was higher among women, it was higher
still among those with learning difficulties. Six of the seven women with
learning difficulties had been victims: four from violence at the hands of
their father (three) and/or step-parent (two), and four from sexual abuse
by someone other than a parent.

Abuse is widely regarded as a manifestation of parental inadequacy
on the part of mothers and fathers with learning difficulties (Dowdney
and Skuse, 1993). Levels of reported abuse among the now-adult children in this study were high and at first sight this finding seems to
support such an interpretation. Closer examination, however, points to
the need for caution. Very few parents with learning difficulties were
themselves directly responsible for abusing their children. Most abuse
was committed by fathers or step-parents without learning difficulties.
The highest incidence of abuse occurred among women with learning
difficulties at the hands of people other than their parents, and what
evidence there is suggests that this group is vulnerable to exploitation
whether their parents have learning difficulties or not (Sobsey, 1994;
Turk and Brown, 1992, 1993). The only safe conclusion seems to be
that women with learning difficulties often become involved with
abusive partners.

Physical maltreatment and sexual exploitation were not the only
forms of abuse experienced by people in the study. They also met with

institutional discrimination and with oppressive treatment from officials of all sorts. (Chapter 9 develops and explores the notion of system abuse as a misuse of power by bureaucratic agencies and their front-line representatives.) On top of all this, most people in the study were affected by victimisation or harassment directed against them personally or their parents and family. Seventeen people reported having been the butt of insults, taunting and mockery serious enough to constitute verbal abuse. There were no differences on this score between people with and without learning difficulties or between men and women. Twelve people said they can remember having to move house – some several times – in order to escape persecution in their homes and neighbourhoods. Similar numbers reported persistent intimidation from neighbours, bullying, being picked on in the street, damage to property and personal injury. Such happenings were generally recounted with the same flat affect as was given to accounts of beatings, rape and incest. It was as if people had become so inured to random cruelty that they had come to accept it as part of their lot. For some their home provided a sanctuary from the evil that lurked outside. For others family life just mirrored the goings on in a nasty world.

Relationships and supports outside the family

The presence of external supports that reward individuals' competencies and bolster their sense of self-esteem is known to be an important factor in helping people through an otherwise difficult childhood (Garmezy, 1991; Werner, 1989). We tried to assess the strength of people's external support systems as children using their own accounts of their relationships outside the family and of their participation and involvement in activities outside the home.

Again working from people's own life stories, a supportive network of relations was taken to be indicated by a combination of having a number of school friends; friends in the neighbourhood; helpful neighbours; a valued service worker; good institutional supports; and at least one supportive adult outside the family. By contrast, a limited or weak network was taken to be indicated by stories telling of a lonely and isolated childhood; bad influences in children's homes; poor institutional supports; and unhappy experiences of dealings with service workers. Participation and involvement outside the home were rated positively where people had lived in a small community; used to pop into other people's houses; were invited to parties and celebrations; attended mainstream schooling; had a job; belonged to local clubs or were active in societies and voluntary organisations. Contra-indications were taken to be frequent changes of school; victimisation in the community; institutional living; residence on a large, impersonal estate; irregular employment; and lack of spare-time activities.

Few people had experienced a supportive environment outside their family. In twenty cases the number of positive sources of support was exceeded by the number of contra-indications. Only five people notched up half or more of the variables used to indicate the presence of supports outside the home, whereas twelve people exceeded the same proportion of negative factors. People with learning difficulties were much less likely to find sources of support in the wider community and much more likely to meet with experiences that undermine the ability to cope. There were no differences in this respect between men and women. An example of someone who enjoyed a predominantly supportive environment is given by Adam Lloyd whose story is presented at the beginning of this chapter. Kerry Sutton shows the flip side of the coin.

Kerry Sutton

Kerry has a physical impairment affecting her legs and spine and finds it painful to stand or walk for long. Her parents divorced when she was seven and she continued to live with her mother, brother and older sister. For many years the family were forced to move from house to house to avoid harassment from local youths. She attended a special school because of her disabilities and spent three years in two children's homes. She also lived for a time with foster parents. After leaving school she remained at home until she was seventeen before starting at a further education college. After nine months, she decided to leave and has been unemployed at home for the last ten years. Kerry has no friends and rarely goes out of the house.

Kitty Simpson was one of the few people with learning difficulties who experienced something approaching a supportive external network:

Kitty Simpson

Kitty lives with her mother. Her father walked out when she was nine years old and she has not had any contact with him since. She and her mum have lived in their present home a long time and the next-door neighbours have always given her mum help with such things as shopping, cutting the grass and by just popping in to see she's all right. Kitty too has a close relationship with these neighbours. She sees them as her second family and calls their two daughters her special sisters. She and her mum have also made friends at the church which they attend regularly. Kitty's horizons have been broadened recently by her attendance at a further education college. This has led to her doing voluntary work in a nursery and an old people's home, and to her going out on social nights to a large sports centre with her college course group.

Research has shown that adequate social supports play a crucial role in fostering resilience in children (see chapter 5) and in sustaining parental competence and family functioning (Booth and Booth, 1994c; Tymchuk, 1992). Few of the now-adult children in this study had the resources of an enabling environment to draw on. Most experienced the world as an unforgiving place all too ready to fasten on to their vulnerabilities. Rather than providing succour the community more often added to their troubles. Against this background, their difficulties cannot all be heaped on to their parents or their family. A finger must be pointed at a society too quick to scapegoat its weakest members.

ADULT IDENTITIES

It is time to return to the question we posed at the start of this chapter. How successfully have the people in our study, born and brought up in a family headed by at least one parent with learning difficulties, managed the transition to adulthood?

Adulthood is a complex and slippery notion. As Jenkins (1989) observes, it refers to 'a phase of the life-course marked by an imprecise threshold'. Adulthood itself is not a clear-cut status but a bundle of identities – worker, wife or husband, householder, parent etc. – the acquisition of which is usually accomplished serially (if at all) at different chronological ages, and influenced by a range of sociological variables including social class, gender, ethnicity and disability. The boundaries between childhood and these different aspects of adulthood are blurred, shifting and hard to define. From this point of view, it may be more appropriate to talk about a range of transitions to a variety of different 'adulthoods'.

Hutson and Jenkins (1989) offer a way through this maze. Adulthood, they suggest, involves both *being* and *doing*. On the one hand, it is 'an officially defined identity' bestowed legally and administratively by the state and bound up with the notion of citizenship as a status conferring rights and duties. On the other hand, it is 'a repertoire of appropriate behaviour': in order to be treated like an adult an individual must in turn behave in certain socially approved ways. Though analytically distinct, the citizenship and performance dimensions of adulthood are wrapped up together in everyday life.

People with learning difficulties are still denied many of those aspects of adulthood associated with full citizenship. They may be deemed incapable of voting. The existing law relating to decision-making embodies 'no coherent concept of their status' (Law Commission, 1991). Their 'reproductive rights' are widely honoured only in the breach (Booth and Booth, 1995; Petchesky, 1979). The hold they exercise on their parental rights is fragile and tenuous at best (Booth and Booth, 1994c, 1996a, 1996b). As victims of crime, men and women with learning difficulties are not treated equally under the law. There is no crime of rape against a woman with learning difficulties (only 'unlawful sexual intercourse'). Men with learning difficulties are 'physically abused' where others are assaulted (Williams, 1995). In these and other ways, people with learning difficulties are officially defined as less than fully adult. One-half of the people in our study had learning difficulties. Their stories were replete with examples of the impact of this sort of discrimination in their daily lives. However, these problems of growing older without growing up are not related to their parentage. They are common to all people with learning difficulties irrespective of their family of origin. Equally, in the case of people without learning difficulties, their assumption of an official identity as adults is relatively unproblematic. For this reason, we shall concentrate the remarks that follow on the performance dimension of adulthood which, involving as it does people's behaviour and their relationships, might reasonably be expected to be influenced by their upbringing and their experience of family life.

Following Kiernan (1986), Morrow and Richards (1996) identify five changes in the transition to adulthood that provide a useful template for thinking about and gauging the experience of the people in our study: leaving school; leaving home; becoming a couple; becoming a parent; and assuming the role of an adult consumer in the marketplace.

Leaving school

The past two decades have seen big changes in the pattern of transition from school into the labour market. In the mid-1970s, over half the population left school at sixteen and most moved into full-time work. Unemployment levels in this age group were low. During the 1980s the youth labour market collapsed. Increasingly, young people remained in education or training, delaying the entry into work or unemployment. The effects of social class differences ensured that unqualified young people were more likely to come from manual backgrounds and to be unemployed. Young disabled people are almost twice as likely to be un-employed. Research has shown that 'achieving independence through employment is an unlikely prospect for most disabled people before their mid-twenties, if at all' (Hirst and Baldwin, 1994). Families and kin networks have been found to play a key part in supporting young people in the transition from school, both in terms of their influence on young people's expectations and aspirations, and in terms of access to resources such as information and contacts.

There was no evidence that the now-adult children without learning difficulties in our study were disadvantaged in making the transition from school by their family background, other than might be expected as a result of their social class and their residence in geographically depressed areas. Although most of the men left school without qualifi-cations, they had also succeeded in the main at keeping themselves in jobs. While most of the women did not have paid employment, the reasons were bound up with ill-health or domestic commitments and reflected the somewhat more complex relationship between gender and labour market participation.

Disability is a major barrier to employment, and people with intel-lectual disabilities are even less likely than people with a physical impairment to find paid work in real jobs (Hirst, 1987). Not surpris-ingly, therefore, like most of their peers, none of the men and women with learning difficulties were in work. There was nothing to differen-tiate their post-school experience from that of other people with learning difficulties except perhaps that fewer were receiving traditional adult day services and a higher proportion were attending Further Education colleges.

Leaving home

A total of thirteen of the thirty people in our study were still living in the parental home. Nine of this group had learning difficulties: two of the rest were disabled and two were the youngest women in the study.

Leaving home is something of a selection process, structured by the operation of the education system, labour market and housing market (Jones, 1995), in which class, gender, ethnicity and disability all interact to influence the age at which people make the break into independent living. Berrington and Murphy (1994) point out that, at later ages, those remaining at home tend to be those who are permanently disabled, on very low incomes or unemployed. The data from our study are consistent with the outcomes from just such a selection process. The only qualification is that the women with learning difficulties were twice as likely as the men to have set up their own home, primarily because they are more likely than men with learning difficulties to find a partner to share it with them.

The transition to coupledom

Sexual maturity is publicly affirmed by the passage into coupledom. There is a suggestion in the literature on parents with learning difficulties that their children might have difficulty in forming and maintaining such relationships because of an emotionally starved childhood. In fact, the only people without learning difficulties who had not had a long-term relationship were those with some form of impairment or who were still quite young and living with their parents. About one in three had experienced the break-up of a long-term partnership – although this proportion is not out of line with rates of dissolution in the wider society, especially among poor families where money problems place an additional strain on relationships (Kempson, 1996; National Children's Home, 1992).

None of the men with learning difficulties had negotiated the transition to coupledom, but three of the seven women had married (one of whom was now divorced). Lack of opportunity, lack of autonomy and active opposition are some of the factors that inhibit the formation of intimate relationships by people with learning difficulties. Evidence suggests that most remain emotionally dependent on their families well into their adult years (Flynn and Hirst, 1992). Families play an important role in shaping young people's ideas about their sexuality, especially in the case of those with learning difficulties who generally miss out on the sources of information available to others. In this context, our study suggests the possibility that, for women with learning difficulties at least, having a mother with learning difficulties may serve as a positive role model.

The transition to parenthood

All the people who were or had been married had children of their own except one of the women with learning difficulties. No-one had had a child outside of marriage. This pattern of child-rearing shows a close adherence to conventional social norms which construct parenthood as a stage in adult development following marriage and homemaking. None of the children of those without learning difficulties had been admitted to care. Both the mothers with learning difficulties have had their children removed. For people with learning difficulties, making the transition to parenthood involves more than just having children. It also means establishing the right to rear them.

Becoming an adult consumer

Morrow and Richards (1996) suggest that 'the establishment of financial independence from one's family of origin and the concomitant ability to become an adult consumer' is an important aspect of the construction of individual adult identity. According to Jones and Wallace (1992) consumption 'can be a source of power, social status and identity even without occupational status'. For those without learning difficulties in our study, their position in this respect was compromised only by the pinching effects of poverty. The situation of the men and women with learning difficulties was different. Disability is known to be a factor that increases financial dependency and reduces consumption power. Hirst and Baldwin (1994) conclude that severely disabled people are 'especially disadvantaged in achieving a degree of financial independence'. Likewise, Flynn and Hirst (1992) found that the financial aspirations of the young people with learning difficulties they surveyed had still to be realised whether in relation to the amount or control of their money. Almost a third of those over eighteen said they never spent their own money without prior permission. There is confirmation of these findings from our study. Few people, even the married women with learning difficulties, controlled their own money. Almost always there was someone in the background – a parent in the case of the younger ones, a husband or a support worker in the case of those living independently – who controlled the purse strings.

Overview

We set out to examine in this section how the people in our study coped with the transition to adulthood conceived as 'a set of practical accomplishments' (Hutson and Jenkins, 1989) encapsulated in the processes of change and development outlined above. Two broad conclusions are justified on the evidence of people's life stories recounted in interview.

In establishing an adult status for themselves in society the men and women without learning difficulties experienced no problems of a type or magnitude sufficient to distinguish them from other people coming from the same socio-economic background.

The situation was somewhat different in the case of the men and women with learning difficulties. Many experienced problems in negotiating the steps into adulthood, especially the men. The women seemed to find it a little easier to slot into some aspects of the traditional female role, especially in the area of establishing emotional relationships outside their family of origin. Flynn and Hirst (1992) suggest that the acquisition of an adult status 'may be postponed indefinitely' for many young people with learning difficulties. This does not seem to be supported by our data – especially, again, in the case of the women. Indeed, there is a suggestion, worth following up with more research, that growing up with a parent or parents with learning difficulties may have a plus side for children with learning difficulties, perhaps because less is made of their limitations within the family.

Chapter 5

Risk, resilience and competence

Resilience refers to the ability to cope with lives filled with difficulty (Begun, 1993; Poulsen, 1993). Rutter (1987) defines it as 'the positive pole of individual variations in people's response to stress and adversity'. Under high-risk conditions, the resilient overcome where the vulnerable succumb (Werner, 1989). Resilience is fostered or enhanced by protective factors which ameliorate an individual's response to risk (Mrazek and Mrazek, 1987). This chapter examines the sources of resilience in the lives of our subjects on the basis of their own narrative reconstruction of their experience as children and young adults.

DOMAINS OF RESILIENCE

Most research so far in this field has adopted a predictive approach that has attempted to identify the protective factors leading to resilience in terms of cause-and-effect relationships between earlier events and later developments (Cohler, 1987). By contrast, we follow a narrative or interpretive approach that seeks to understand how people make sense of their past and how they reflect upon their own experience as the source of their vulnerability or resilience. As Cohler (1987) has observed, little is still known about the manner in which people reflect upon their own past in order 'to create a narrative that renders adversity coherent in terms of experienced life history'. This chapter is an attempt to address this challenge by identifying the protective factors present in people's life stories that appear to have served as a counterweight to the risks inherent in their upbringing.

The research literature suggests that the protective factors shielding high-risk children fall into three interrelated domains: personal characteristics, family characteristics, and the characteristics of the individual's wider social environment and external support system. Werner (1989), for example, concludes that:

> Three types of protective factors emerge from our analyses of the developmental course of high-risk children from infancy to adulthood: 1) dispositional attributes of the individual, such as activity level and sociability, at least average intelligence, competence in communication skills (language, reading), and an internal locus of control; 2) affectional ties within the family that provide emotional support in times of stress, whether from a parent, sibling, spouse or mate; and 3) external support systems, whether in school, at work, or church, that reward the individual's competencies and determination, and provide a belief system by which to live.

We have used this same framework to analyse the content of our informants' narratives.

Personal protective factors

According to Rutter (1987), the available evidence suggests that 'it is protective to have a well established feeling of one's own worth as a person together with a confidence that one can cope successfully with life's challenges'. Three qualities appeared to be linked to the presence of such feelings in the personal narratives of the people in our study:

- *Sociability* – as revealed through a friendly and personable disposition, good communication skills, conventional looks and manner, good physical and mental health, not having learning difficulties, a non-violent nature, and socially acceptable behaviour.
- *Responsiveness to others* – as revealed through the capacity to maintain close and/or intimate relationships, expressions of love and feelings of responsibility for family members, and protectiveness towards the parent(s) with learning difficulties.
- *Successful task accomplishment* – such as participation in voluntary activities, taking on responsibilities, having outside interests, being good at sports and, especially for people with learning difficulties, being able to read and write.

There were a few individual characteristics, not necessarily socially desirable, that did not easily fit into this listing but, for some people, seemed to contribute to their resilience, including being rebellious, outspoken, independent-minded and ambitious.

Protective mechanisms within the family

Resilient children are:

> more likely to come from home environments characterised by warmth, affection, emotional support, and clear-cut and reasonable structures and limits. If parents are not able to provide this kind of positive climate, the presence of other family members can serve this function.
>
> (Brooks, 1994)

Similar factors were evident in the personal stories of those adults in our study who spoke positively of their own childhood, and tended to be missing in the narratives of those who did not. Three characteristics of the family and home environment in particular appeared to contribute to greater resilience in the face of risk:

- *Warmth and mutuality* – as revealed by, for example, feelings of having been loved as a child, being a wanted child, experiencing fair and effective discipline, not being abused, and sharing holidays and other activities as a family.
- *Stability* – as indicated by, for example, having two natural parents, one parent without learning difficulties, an absence of separations or the death of a close relative, and a parent or parents alive throughout childhood.
- *Security* – as marked by, for example, having grandparents who live near, having a supportive uncle or aunt at home, having a single parent but living in the same household with grandparents, having a large supportive extended family, coming from a financially secure home and having parents who can manage money.

Protective social supports

A key feature noted in the literature for nurturing resilience is the presence of external supports that reinforce the child's and family's competence in coping under pressure. A close reading of our informants' life stories points to two aspects of the wider social environment that seem to be important as buffers against stress:

- *Supportive relationships* – as shown, for example, by some combination of having a number of school friends, friends in the neighbourhood, helpful neighbours, a valued service worker, good institutional supports from agencies such as a school, church, health centre etc., and at least one supportive person outside the family.

* *Participation and involvement* – as indicated by, for example, some combination of living in a small, tightly knit community, popping in to people's houses, holding and going to parties and celebrations, mainstream schooling, having a job or some sort of access to ordinary workplace opportunities, belonging to local clubs, such as the darts team, or being active in societies, such as a group of bird-watchers, and organisations such as the local church.

A compensatory model

The protective factors outlined above may be missing for some people, or they may change over time, or they may be insufficient to buttress the individual against the pressures bearing on them. The balance between the stresses that heighten vulnerability and the protective factors that enhance resilience varies for different individuals and at different points in people's lives. Werner (1989), for example, notes that as disadvantage and the number of stressful life events accumulate, so more protective factors are needed to ensure a positive outcome. Such a compensatory model of the interaction between resilience and risk (McIntyre *et al.*, 1990) suggests that competence is maintained where the protective factors outweigh the risks and undermined where they do not. From this perspective, resilience, and for that matter competence, is better viewed as a process determined by the impact of an individual's life experiences than as a fixed attribute of the person.

The next section focuses on the personal narratives of two people in our study in order to show this process at work in the context of people's lives.

RESILIENCE AND THE LIFE COURSE

The following two narratives have been selected from the stories of informants in the study in order to represent the two ends of the continuum from vulnerability to resilience and to show that people's destiny is not fixed by having a mother (or father) with learning difficulties.

A vulnerable life: Chris Sutton's story

Chris Sutton is 26 years old. When first interviewed Chris was living in a tenth floor council flat on the outskirts of a large city. Most days he would visit his parents who lived two bus journeys away. By the third interview he had moved in with them and his disabled sister, Kerry, owing to the sudden onset of a paralysis in his right arm. His parents live in a three-bedroom house on a council estate in a small town. They were happy there although both of them are beginning to find the steep hills a problem. Mr and Mrs Sutton divorced eighteen years ago and Chris and Kerry spent most of their lives with their mother who has learning difficulties. Mr and Mrs Sutton re-married last year. They also have an elder daughter, Jane, who is married and lives away.

Still close to family

Ill-health

Break-up of parents' marriage

Mother with learning difficulties

The family is only friendly with two people in the neighbourhood: one of whom is out all day and the other does child-minding. To some extent Kerry's disability has disabled the whole family. They can't and won't go out and leave her alone and she is unable to walk far. They have no car but they are on the telephone.

Social isolation

Disabled sibling

Lack of mobility

Chris is slim, with longish fair hair combed forward over his forehead. He has a curved spine and a disability in his right shoulder and arm. Dressed in jeans and a dark jumper, he is easygoing, polite and friendly. Although unemployed at present, he has had various part-time jobs as a cleaner. He is a sensitive and caring person and helps his mother regularly with the shopping. He sometimes also does the washing, hoovering and cleaning for her.

Looks different

Responsive to others

Sense of duty

Chris was only six years old when his mother and father separated. 'Mostly,' he says, 'it were gambling and drinking that my mum and dad split up for.' He remembers his parents arguing a lot too and how his mother once hit his father over the head with a frying pan and threatened him with a meat cleaver.

Chronic family discord

Much of Chris' childhood was clouded by violence and fear. Local children would abuse him physically and verbally in the street and at school: 'Oh they were kicking me, pulling my hair, cutting my hair. . . . Well, there were a kid and he put me through school railings. . . . I mean I once got my clothes all chucked into shower and I had to go home in absolute complete wet clothes.' He was also physically attacked by his older sister who has since gone on to abuse her own five children, three of whom are now in care.

Victimisation

Sibling with behaviour problem

Mrs Sutton recalled having lived in places where their lives were turned into a nightmare by local teenagers who used to pinch the washing off the line, bang on the windows and doors, shout abuse, and push fireworks through the letterbox. 'I got police but police wouldn't do nowt.' One night Chris had his nose broken by a gang of youths. Even after they moved house, 'all of a sudden these gangs of teenagers started on us for no apparent reason'. His mother eventually had a nervous breakdown.

Constant harassment

Parental mental ill-health

Mrs Sutton and her three children moved house seven times, mainly in a vain attempt to escape the constant victimisation. The one place they really liked they couldn't afford: 'It were a lovely place that, it were just bills all the time because it were all electric.' All his childhood Chris recalls the family having difficulty managing on their low income. They finally moved to their present house and for ten years have felt safe.

Frequent changes of residence

Poverty

Chris began his education at a mainstream school but at the age of seven he was transferred to a special school because of his behaviour. By the time he was thirteen, he was under a psychiatrist and attending a special psychiatric unit.

Segregated schooling/ separated from peers

Chris' mental health problems began when he started eating an excessive number of chocolate bars. He became 'disturbed and overactive with fits and violent outbursts'. He was given a brain scan and a body scan. 'I were breaking things, putting table upside down, barricading doors, doing all

Mental health problems

sorts. . . . I spent four months in there having different tests and that, having different fluids taken out of me.' As he now quietly reflects, 'if we'd known it were Mars bars we could have stopped that years ago'. Even so he felt content in the unit and became quite attached to one of the nurses while he was there.

Chris remained overactive and was given sleeping tablets as he got older. He is no longer prescribed these tablets as he once overdosed after his uncle had died. Since then he has tried other ways to kill himself by 'jumping off a bridge, trying to chuck myself in front of cars, trying to cut my wrists'. 'It's mostly with depression . . . because I get that low and I get that fed up.'

Depression

He disliked school mainly because of the bullying he endured throughout his time there. He had problems with reading and writing and found his teachers unhelpful. He left at fifteen. On his last day he punched a female teacher who had tried to stop him leaving. This action, he felt, had prevented him from being accepted at a further education college. He subsequently drifted into a variety of part-time jobs interspersed with long periods of unemployment.

Lack of achievement

No support from teachers

Sporadic employment

His mother and father had started their married life with Mr Sutton's parents where they lived until after their first child was born. Both sets of grandparents were alive at this time and lived close to one another. There were also numerous uncles and aunts. However, within a few years of moving out into their own home, the marriage had ended. Chris remembers how he and Kerry took the news. 'I know she cried when they splitted up. Me, I wouldn't talk. I wouldn't do owt, you know. I used to get a fork and stick it into my belly button. . . . When they split up it seemed weird. Because, I mean, they weren't there arguing. There were only my mum there. It just seemed to be one empty shell.'

Additional caretakers

Availability of kin

Low self-worth

Father absent

Insecurity

After Chris' father left, his mother received no maintenance money and very little help with the three children. Chris did as much as he could from a

Lack of support for family

very early age, washing the pots, cleaning and even doing the washing. He also helped look after Kerry, and still does. Once a year they would go to Skegness and stay in their grandparent's caravan. Chris enjoyed these times. Looking back, he never felt he had missed out on anything as a child. He thinks he was mostly happy.

Other-regarding

Family togetherness

Positive outlook

Chris moved out of the family home when he was seventeen, and for a while lived in a hostel for homeless young people. 'I were wanting my own space you know. But I felt really homesick for the first two months.' For the next five years he had a bedsit, and then a flat next door to a drug dealer. He left this flat to move back home. Chris feels he has always had a close relationship with his mother and recalls being cuddled by her, although that has stopped since he became an adult. He sees his dad differently, 'I mean I've never considered him as a dad. It's a bit of a relief for him to come back into the family. It's like him taking over, giving me a rest point. I mean what makes my mum happy, that's all right to me.'

Self-sufficient

Poor environment

Close affectional ties

Positive mother-child relationship

When the children were small the family had received help from the paternal grandparents who had looked after the oldest daughter, Jane, for a few years, and also helped them out financially. Otherwise there had been little support from elsewhere. A social worker had been attached to the family after Kerry was born but Chris feels they 'had not done owt . . . it's just a waste of time'.

Practical support from extended family

Service worker not valued

His happiest memory as a child is playing with a gang of local children: 'Playing Cowboys and Indians . . . going all round back fields. . . . We used to go down to shops with a bit of spending money . . . and buy some sweets.' He was good at athletics; it was one of the only things he liked doing at school. 'I were one of top runners in our school.' He had a few close friends as a child but none as a teenager and he has made no friends since he left school. No-one ever came round his house to play.

Loss of friendships and peer relation-ships as adult

Chris thinks of himself as being very close to his extended family: 'Oh yes, we're very close, yes. We've all got us own way of getting in touch with each other.' But the extent of contact is limited: 'Well, we do see them now and again in town. . . . We don't actually visit them, or owt like that, because it'd be a bit too much because there's that many of us.' Nobody comes to visit them.

Emotional ties with extended family

Weak contiguous bonds

Chris has mixed thoughts about his future. Sometimes he wishes he could move south and start a new life. At other times he is haunted by a recurring dream of his own funeral. He believes he will be dead by the time he is thirty-three.

A month after the last interview, Chris suffered what turned out to be his second stroke. The first had gone undiagnosed by his GP. He is totally paralysed down one side and both his speech and mental ability have been affected. He is sleeping downstairs at his parents house. With his father too ill to help, the job of looking after Chris and Kerry, who has to be taken to the toilet and is still incontinent at times, now falls entirely on their mother. They are waiting to be rehoused but have been told this could take at least six months.

Lack of institutional support for family in crisis

A resilient life: Martin Riddick's story

Risk factors/ Protective factors

Martin Riddick is forty two years old. He lives in a one-bedroom flat owned by a housing association with his elder son, Graham, aged sixteen. Graham has laid claim to the bedroom, while his dad sleeps on the settee. Martin is looking to buy his own house. He works shifts as a support worker for a Community Health project for people with learning difficulties and also does other work in his trade as a roofer. Since leaving school he has tried his hand at a variety of jobs including work as a hotel porter and voluntary work with a young man who has Down's syndrome. His younger son, Christopher, aged ten, still lives with Martin's ex-wife who is now remarried.

Own home

Regular employment

Marriage breakdown

Martin is short and slight with longish dark hair greying at the sides. He speaks in a quiet voice and his manner is open and hospitable. His marriage ended seven years ago and for the last three years he has been friendly with a woman who herself has been married before and has children of her own.

Conventional appearance

New stable relationship

As a small child Martin lived with his mother, who had learning difficulties, and his father at his maternal grandparents' house. 'I think the reason why they got married is the fact that I think I was on the way. In them days it was the done thing.' Also living with the grandparents were his mum's brother, who remained there all his life, and his mum's younger sister and her husband. His mum also had another married sister. Martin's two brothers were born after his parents were allocated their own house.

Mother with learning difficulties

Tightly knit extended family

Plenty of attention in infancy

Eldest child

His father had held a number of regular jobs. After he left the army he worked in the steel industry, before becoming a long-distance lorry driver and later a bus driver. His mum too had worked even after Martin was born: first as a buffer in a cutlery firm, and then in a sweet factory. They had met one night at a public dance in the town hall. His father had attended Catholic schools but his mum went to special school. Unlike other families in their neighbourhood, the Riddicks had owned a car when Martin was young, although they were not on the phone.

Financially secure early childhood

Mother in steady employment

Mobile and relatively well-off

Martin had enjoyed life at home with his grandparents and at his first school. It was when his parents moved into their own house that things became more difficult. Martin was eight and his brother, Keith, was two when the family moved to the other side of the city. Four years later a third brother, Damien, was born. From this time onwards things started to become strained at home. 'I know that my dad had had affairs because I know that I've got another half-sister who's probably a few months younger than me that lives in Liverpool.' His mum and dad would argue quite a bit and occasionally they would separate only to be reunited soon after.

Happy start to life

Loss of additional carers

Children spaced apart

Family discord

'Sometimes it got really bad and my middle brother, Keith, he were starting to be very nervous.' When Martin was about fourteen his parents split up for good and were divorced. 'Knowing that it weren't going to get better, it was probably the best. But saying that, it didn't help the fact that my mum were like she were, it didn't help me, Keith and Damien.' His dad disappeared out of the area for a few years and it was only later that Martin learned he had gone to live with another woman. The two of them later married and had two girls, Martin's half-sisters.

Parents' divorce

Positive outlook

Loss of contact with father

Martin's mother was devastated by the break-up of her marriage and, seeking comfort, she took up with a series of men. The neighbours began to gossip. Martin heard the talk 'not so much through them but by people at school who were their sons and daughters. I didn't like that.' Martin also did a lot of babysitting at this time when his mum wanted to go out with a boyfriend. 'I always tried to get on with them for my mum's sake. I knew that she were lonely.' These relationships affected Martin and his brothers greatly. He would occasionally confront her, 'I'd say, it's not fair for us, people gossiping. And that would probably cause friction between me and my mum.' At one point she really let herself go and ended up having a nervous breakdown. She was admitted to a long-stay psychiatric hospital where she remained for a year while Martin and his brothers went to live with their grandparents. 'We never visited my mum while she were in hospital because it used to upset her ... or, as my grandma said, it would upset her when we were leaving. Because when they fetched her it were a real struggle to get her in the ambulance, to take her away.'

Emotional insecurity

Sensitive to other's needs

Sense of responsibility

Parental mental illness and separation

Additional caretakers besides mother

Martin's mother received no maintenance from his father and the family suffered as a result. 'I found that when my dad did leave and money were short, my mum got help to buy uniform but, like, when it wore out, we had to buy things probably what didn't quite fit and I found then I started getting noticed, like, because I looked a bit untidy. So from fourteen, my last two years were a nightmare because I were getting picked on, bullied in some cases, getting into

Financial hardship

Victimisation

trouble, getting into fights. So it's like the only way out, to stop them talking, is probably giving someone a smack, which obviously isn't the right way of doing it, as you find out. It just gets you into trouble, it pushes you further away from neighbours. Probably the ideal system would be to have gone up and said, look, you know the situation my mum's in, do you mind not talking about it.'

Maturity through self-knowledge

From the age of five until he was fifteen, Martin spent every weekend with his grandparents. It was here that his close friends lived. His dearest memories are of his childhood Saturdays. They always followed the same pattern: 'Saturday was always a good time. Pictures in the morning, came home from pictures, had my dinner, then from pictures played with my mates all day and then we all went to the football match. At night, we'd come home from football match, had us tea and we used to go to pub with my grandma and granddad and my Auntie Doris. I used to sit in the corridor on a bench with some pop and a bag of crisps. It made my day.'

Close relationship with adults outside the home providing security and stability

Strong peer friendships

Martin attended three schools in his life but only suffered trouble and unhappiness at the senior school. He missed a lot of time at school by pretending to be poorly. Apart from being the butt of cruel remarks about his mother and their poverty, Martin had dyslexia. His difficulties went unrecognised by his teachers and he struggled with his lessons and failed his 'O' levels. Dyslexia was only diagnosed later on in life when he went back to college to take some GCSEs, successfully passing in maths, English, sociology and law. He says he still enjoyed some aspects of his schooldays mainly because he was good at sport, especially football and swimming.

Poor school attendance

Specific learning difficulties

Sense of self-efficacy and self-esteem

It was after his father left that Martin became aware of the extent of his mother's learning difficulties. 'We never really had to think about mum because my dad did it all anyway. I suppose we did know, but it never really dawned on us how it would affect the family if anything happened to my dad.'

His dad had even prepared meals before he went off to work ready for when the boys came home from school. Martin's mum couldn't read letters, notes from school or claims for rent arrears and she found managing the domestic budget an almost impossible task. Martin gradually assumed more and more responsibility for running the house. When she received her benefits the family would dine 'like princes' on chops and steak for a few days until the money ran out when it would be jam or dripping sandwiches or meat paste.

Loss of principal carer

Parent with learning difficulties left on own

Advanced self-help skills

Martin and his brothers decided they would have to do something about the situation. 'We've always been close, me and my brothers. It weren't like, "I'm taking over so you do what I say." It were like, best work together. They were really supportive.' Martin always talked things over with his brothers and then presented their suggestions to their mother. They would go shopping with her and advise on what foodstuffs to choose, suggesting cheaper meats such as sausage and liver.

Shared values – sense of togetherness

'When my dad first left I probably felt, like, I'm man of house now and I probably felt I were getting a bit clever. But, I think, once I saw how it affected my mum and how it upset her . . . then my aunties said, look, man of house don't need to be going off like you are doing, get to grips. And then I realised that I were getting bad, and I thought, yes, you're not helping situation at all. I think from that time on, it were a case of we'll all pull together. So we did like grow up very quick.'

Matured through self-knowledge

Internal locus of control

When Mrs Riddick decided they should move nearer to her own parents, Martin's grandmother and two aunties provided the extra support the family needed. 'It's about ten minutes walk to any of relatives. They'd help out best they could.' His mum also knew quite a few of the neighbours 'who weren't just talking (they) were helping out a lot'. The only formal support the family received was a bundle of second-hand toys delivered by social services at Christmas.

Availability of kin

Support from neighbours

Lack of formal support

Discipline in Martin's life was fairly strict. His mum and dad would keep him in check with a swift slap on the arm and his aunties would slap him on the legs. Sometimes 'if I'd been a bit clever and my dad had been on nights, I remember getting a few real hidings from him'. But afterwards 'it used to be all apologies'. Occasionally he would be kept in or sent to his bedroom. His teachers at school were much more brutal. Punishment for lateness was a detention, but for bad work or behaviour it could be a ruler across the knuckles, a slipper on the bottom (once when he was only wearing swimming trunks) or the cane on both hands. He was once slapped across the face for poor work although he now knows the problem was his dyslexia. 'What made it more painful, it were by a teacher what I really liked.' Martin, however, was treated no differently from the rest of his classmates. 'You weren't one of the boys unless you got it. If you got caught then you got a punishment. If you didn't get caught, you got away with it. It was just something you accepted really.'

Fair and effective discipline

Structure and rules in household

Positive attitude to authority

Martin has only once been in trouble with the police. 'Went down town with some friends and something happened and then these lads saw me following day at the football match and it turned into a bit of a fight like. We both got arrested. I got fined £70 and a suspended sentence for twelve months on good behaviour. I got more of a reaction from my grandma and my aunties than I did from my mum. It were a case of, "What you doing, you're not like this, look at shame you're bringing your dad and your mum." It made me feel right tiny.'

Strong moral guidance and authority

Martin left school at fifteen and went straight into a job. For the first time in his life, he was able to buy the clothes he wanted, and sometimes for Keith too. 'I'm not making out to be good like, but occasionally you could say, "Well I know what I went through, I'll get you a pair of trousers."' He never resented having to help Keith out: 'What I would have resented more is kids giving Keith a hard time at school.'

No period of unemployment after leaving school

Financial independence

Responsive to others

Martin always had close friends at school but he never invited anyone back to his house because of the sad state of the old furniture and the general untidiness. 'I didn't really want them to see it because my mum weren't a great person to keep the house tidy.' He never blamed his mother though 'because I knew it weren't down to her, I knew that she'd tried everything in her power to make everything all right'. Today Martin feels, 'We've all come out of it probably better for it, me, Keith and Damien. Probably responsibility were there at an early age. Where if the money were there you'd probably think, can I have this and they'd probably let us have it. I know what it's like not to have it. So you're more responsible with your money and probably more tolerant with people that are just down on their luck.'

Strong sense of loyalty and protectiveness towards mother

Positive self-concept

During his late teens his mother finally settled down with a new partner, although she never re-married. Martin's current relationship brings to mind his own feelings at that time. 'Looking back on my mum, I can imagine what my girlfriend's youngest must be thinking. And it did actually come back . . . now how should I handle this? So I had to really think hard about trying to get a friendship with her.'

Matured through experience

When he was twenty-one, Martin left with some friends to find work in the south of England. Here he eventually met his wife and settled. When their marriage ran into difficulties, they returned to his home town to try and sort things out. Finally they parted and his wife moved back down south.

Marriage breakdown

'I think I've always been lucky and I've always been able to make friends very easy. Probably the hardest time was when my marriage split up and I moved back. Where before you could always call on your friends – because they were single – to go for a pint, now it were a case of, well he's married, he doesn't live here no more and, like, you thought, I'm actually stuck for the first time. It were a case of making friends all over again really . . . night school, getting involved in squash and badminton, getting involved in different activities.'

Sociable

Positive social orientation

He decided to improve his education. 'If I were reading out loud, it were embarrassing more than anything else. And my spelling, I couldn't spell quite simple words. I still do roofing but I just didn't feel like doing just that for the rest of my life, and to get into what I wanted to do I knew that I couldn't do it unless I put myself out to get some qualifications behind me.' He is now reaping the rewards of that hard work and likes nothing better than 'helping people with learning difficulties to make a bit of life for themselves.'

Motivated to improve himself

Personally ambitious

Understanding of others

Martin has always felt close to his mother. 'I always loved my mum, especially when my dad left. I loved her more, well if you can love more, because she were really pining after my dad and you just wanted to hold her and say, "It's all right."' She would hug and kiss him as a child, while his father would occasionally put his arm round his shoulder. He knew his father loved him by how he talked to him and by the way he would sit on his bed at night and relate stories of his days in the army. 'He showed his affection by laughing and joking a lot.' After the break-up of his parents' marriage, he grew distant from his father and didn't see him for a few years. Five years ago his mother died suddenly at the age of sixty-two. Today he still calls round to see his father and step-mother, and enjoys the company of his half-sisters, but he is not close to his father. 'The real people in my life was, like, my mum, my two brothers, and my grandma and granddad and my aunties. I still loved him but not in a close way.'

Positive mother-child relationship

Close affectional ties in early childhood

Renewal of family bonds in adult life

'Sounds a bit rotten but I think we've always been closer to my grandma. I know I have. I think we all have. Because, like, she were always there when we needed her. So when my mum did go into hospital, my grandma and aunties were still there. I think if we were taken away and put into care it would probably be a different story altogether. But the fact that we were living with people we loved, it didn't change a great deal. Yes, I loved my mum to death but, you know, my grandma were like the matriarch of family.'

Mother-substitute available when needed

Secure emotional foundation

'Sometimes I think no, it weren't a happy time, especially at school. But in general, I can think of a lot more people having a worse time. It weren't like getting beatings or, you know. In general, I don't think I fared too bad. I did have a happy childhood.'

Positive attitude to life

Chris Sutton and Martin Riddick have much in common. They both come from families where the parents' marriage broke up leaving a mother with learning difficulties to cope on her own with three children. Their early lives were marked by poverty, under-achievement at school, lack of support from the services and their mother's breakdown under the strain. On the positive side, they both had a father without learning difficulties with whom they maintained contact in later life, a close and protective relationship with their mother, a strong sense of responsibility for the family, and supportive grandparents. At this point, however, the similarities in their stories end. Where Chris is now back living at home with his parents, unemployed, disabled, lonely, depressed and suicidal, Martin is a family man, with his own home, in regular work, full of ambitions and well-integrated in the local community. Coming from much the same background, their lives have taken a very different course. Looked at through the framework presented above, their stories show how the balance between risk and protective factors helped to shape these outcomes. Table 1 highlights some of the key biographical experiences contributing to the differences in their resilience.

The wider significance of this analysis of two personal narratives is in showing how resilience (in the face of risk) and competence (in dealing with the pressures and challenges of living) are not merely natural endowments but are socially produced in the context of people's lives and experience.

Table 1   Dimensions of Resilience

Protective factors	Chris Sutton	Martin Riddick
Personal protective factors:		
Sociability	Unconventional looks, poor mental health and disability, past record of violent behaviour	Good communication skills, capacity to make and maintain friendships, positive social orientation
Responsiveness	No close relationships outside family, low self-esteem	Wide network of relationships (including two children of his own), matured through experience
Task accomplishment	Few achievements aside from being good at sport at school	Leading an independent life with a home of his own, successful return to further education, desire to improve himself, active hobbies
Family factors:		
Warmth and mutuality	Physically abused by elder sister, only a year between each of the	Children spaced 6 years apart, brothers close to each other
Stability	Parents split up when he was aged 6, left home at 17 to live in hostel for homeless	Parents didn't split up until he was aged 14, continuity provided by matriarchal grandmother
Security	Repeated changes of residence, financial hardship throughout childhood, persistent victimisation, younger sister admitted to care	Family comfortably off until father left home, strong sense of place during childhood, lived with grandparents as an infant and again during mother's spell in psychiatric hospital
Social supports:		
Supportive relationships	Lonely and isolated	Long-standing peer friendships as youngster and adolescent, socially engaged as adult
Participation and involvement	Segregated schooling, irregular employment, few contacts in local community	Mainstream schooling, regular employment, range of outside interests and voluntary activities

Chapter 6

Still family
Two sisters talk of growing up with a mother who has learning difficulties

The house stands in a well-maintained row of council properties with neat gardens at the bottom of a long road leading from the bustling market centre of a former mining town. The front room is cosy, modern and comfortable. On the velvet settee sit the two sisters, side by side. Sandra, plumpish with short, streaked blonde hair, neatly styled, wears a long skirt, colourful blouse and has a smiling, open face. Maggie is smaller, slim and dressed in brown jeans and white stretch T-shirt. She smokes as she talks, holding a steady gaze. The dog has been shut in the kitchen.

'I'm Maggie Lewis, I'm twenty-eight. I live here by myself.'

'And I'm Sandra West. I'm thirty-two, married, with one child, a boy, fourteen nearly. I live at Kenwell, six mile away. I live in a bungalow. It's us own, we're buying it. We've been down there fourteen years in October, been buying it about eight years. Two bedroom bungalow. We started off renting it, he let us have it dead cheap. You couldn't buy nowhere what we got it for. We're happy enough there, I mean place, we like. We've got a car and phone as well.'

'We both work at Fox's on packing, in packing department. About eight years now, isn't it Sandra? It's twenty-two hours, evening shifts. And I've also got a collecting job, collecting agent, like debt collecting. That's just, like, at weekends. I've worked at a few places but I've been better on evenings because I used to look after my grandma and that, so I was with her in day.'

'We've always lived here. Been in our family about sixty year, probably over now. And who lived in here when we was little was grandma, granddad, Muriel, our Anna, that's Muriel's younger sister, and then me and Maggie come along and I think . . . had our Anna left when Muriel had our Tracey?'

'Grandma always said Anna got married when Tracey come home. Anna got married then, that's what grandma used to say.'

'Muriel's our mother. But we've never called her mam.'

'This street, it was one of the best, one of best streets.'

'I think it's gone downhill now.'

'Putting people on the street that's right thieves and trouble-makers. Before the only trouble-maker was Muriel. But I remember the neighbours were brilliant. If anybody died you'd see grandma going up, grandma and Joan collecting, you know.'

'Used to have a lot to do with lads an' all next door when we were little. She'd got six lads, Nancy. . . . '

'We all used to play together, all the lads.'

'She used to be ever so nice to us. But she died. She died young. Forty something. They're still next door. Well, Derek is, lads aren't. They've never moved.'

'Here there's a kitchen and a front room, and then you've just got your toilet, pantry and that. Bathroom upstairs and three bedrooms. I know, like, our Anna had a bedroom on her own and Muriel had a bedroom on her own.'

'And grandma had a double bed.'

'Sandra slept in single bed and I slept with grandma. How old was I, Sandra, when I stopped sleeping with grandma? Eleven probably, and I hated that, not sleeping with her. Because I used to always put my arm round her and kiss her, say goodnight, grandma. And I hated not doing, I couldn't see why I shouldn't be sleeping with her. And when I got a bed on my own it were foul. Granddad slept downstairs, he couldn't get upstairs. Granddad worked at pit all his life, didn't he? He used to, couldn't breathe, he got . . . coal dust. Granddad died. His lung collapsed. And I think on death certificate it was that coronary thrombosis, all to do with pit.'

'I can remember we used to play cards with him . . . because we've always been a carding family . . . and we used to play cards with him, and if Maggie used to win, she were a "bloody cheat", you know.'

'But then again I used to do all his wash. He used to have gout an' I used to do his feet for him when I were little. I think because I was a nuisance he used to say, "If anything happens to me I'm coming back to haunt you". And that frightened me . . . it frightened me when granddad died that he were going to come back. We was a handful though, weren't we Sandra? Must have been.'

'He was about seventy-six when he died. Grandma died five year ago.'

'When grandma died Muriel wanted to move out, didn't she? She wasn't satisfied. So where'd she go first, Sandra? Was it Bawtry? She went to Bawtry . . . like a halfway house, wasn't it? And we told them about her – didn't we? – and we all went to meeting and told them, "Oh, she'll be OK, she'll be OK, we can cope." They didn't cope very long with her.'

'They just wanted her out though, didn't they, because she is a nuisance, isn't she?'

'Now there's three people, like, sharing. I think she is, like, the worst one of them, she causes havoc there. But the lady died. . . . Bob's wife . . . he looks after them on his own. She's not far away.'

'Yes, he gets paid for looking after them.'

'Sandra moved out when you were eighteen, didn't you Sandra?'

'When I left home I went to my cousin's, our Linda's home. I don't know, I just wasn't very happy at home with everything. I mean, Maggie, you did used to be a sod, didn't you?'

'Yes. . . . Be honest, I'm not bothered.'

'I went to my cousin's. I was pleased when we got back speaking to grandma because I think that caused ill-feeling – didn't it? – with every-body, when I went to a relation.'

'Didn't you come back when you were pregnant?'

'I come back before that. I think I must have been eighteen and half, because I had William at nineteen and half.'

'Our Tracey's now got a baby of her own. She's twenty-one next month.'

'Well, Tracey's a bit difficult, she's a bit slow.'

'Bit backward.'

'Yes, she's a mother now but she's slow and she's sort of. . . . What would you say, Maggie?'

' . . . Highly strung.'

'Yes, throws a bit of a tantrum. Yes, you know, she's got the age probably of a . . . summat like a thirteen-year-old and she's twenty. I mean, she's grown up more with baby. Baby's lovely.'

' . . . And she looks all right, and you think she's all right, and then, all of a sudden, she'd say something really silly.'

'Yet she's got to have the best for the baby. I mean she come up, she's got a brand new pram-pushchair, hundred and summat pound, hasn't she? Instead of making do with a cheap little buggy . . . no, won't do for our Tracey.'

'She's done quite well. She was offered help by social services, but she wouldn't have it. A boyfriend lives with her.'

'We was there when Muriel brought our Tracey home from hospital. It's twenty year ago. Grandma said she wasn't going to let her bring this last one, our Tracey, home. She said, "I'm not having it now at my age", because, I mean, grandma were getting on, and she wasn't well, and all of a sudden ambulance were there and Muriel were coming out with Tracey.'

'She brought Tracey home. No choice. I mean, when she brought you home, Sandra, grandma thought, "Yes, fair enough." But when they brought me home an' all, they said they wasn't having me, they was letting me be adopted, didn't they? But grandma took one look, she couldn't do it. Soft as owt, weren't she, grandma? She couldn't do it. So then I came along and then Tracey came along . . . she was definitely not having Tracey.'

'Grandma looked after Sandra. But, like, Muriel used to take me out and that to Doncaster and Rotherham. She used to take me to these right dumps, she were a right un for men, so we were aware of who she was and that. First thing I remember. . . . I would imagine it started at school . . . I mean, most things about Muriel is, like, embarrassment of her. We was very embarrassed of her, like we wouldn't bring friends home. Only people, like, who knew her and what she was.'

'From being little, I can always remember, people call her, didn't they? I think it'd be more for me when I was at the second school, between seven and eleven, that it more bothered me then than it did at little school.'

'She was violent at that time.'

'Nasty, swearing.'

'Yes, if anybody spoke to her across road she'd go and smack them one at one time. You know, Anna, her younger sister, I mean if she brought friends home, Muriel'd go for them sometimes.'

'Next minute she'd be right as rain, couldn't do enough for you. . . . '

' . . . You know, say she was sorry and everything. Grandma always gave in to her, always gave in to her. She mollycoddled her, didn't she Sandra?'

'She said she'll never change, it's you that's got to change.'

'I think Muriel were on needles, quite a while ago, wasn't it? Muriel used to have a nurse that come in and give her needles. She used to lie on floor on her back, like, with her eyes at back of head because of these needles. As I grew older I used to say to grandma, "I think she's putting a lot of it on". Every week she'd to have injections. Every week in her bottom. Got her off them. They used to calm her down but they was giving side effects. I mean, they'd just say, "All right, Muriel?", and she'd swear at them, right across street, and then they'd ignore her. And people'll say, "Muriel swore at me!", and I'd just say, "Ignore her next time". Grandma used to get embarrassed as well, always apologising for her, you know. That's just it, you're always having to warn people, aren't you Sandra? If you bring somebody home you have to tell them about her.'

'When it comes to birthdays, mother's day, Christmas, you know, we never, ever miss her out. Even though on a mother's day card I put, 'To Muriel' . . . I won't put "To mum" in it . . . but we never, ever miss her out. And I don't think anybody, you know, nobody really misses her out. And there's a lot of us, a lot of girls in family, and we're all quite close. And I mean she's done summat horrible to everybody.'

'Muriel used to get on at work, didn't she? I mean, you know, she says she's had eight jobs. And she were pretty good. Muriel used to work at Garden Centre, didn't she Sandra? They used to think she were great there. I don't know what she did. McDonalds, I think she worked at McDonalds, you know, serving and things like that. I don't think she'd be on till, she'd just be giving orders out. I think she were laid off or something like that. She was a cleaner at Co-op, where they make plastic bags, because I used to go with her, and you did, didn't you Sandra? Because I remember she liked it, she loved that, that job. She must have been right to get a job down there. People used to say, "That's Muriel, can't do nowt about it", you know. I can remember when she had argument with a woman next door but one, pulling her hair and all lot, fighting, Muriel was. Only a little bit of a thing, and this woman great big. She was frightened of nobody. People were frightened of her.'

'We went to Christchurch school – didn't we Maggie? – and then Maltby Road, and then Hanstead Grange. Maltby Road's a middle school. That's just up top of road. Little school's just over there, the gates only just up main road. Hanstead Grange's about a ten-minute walk, if that. We've always lived here, we've always been here.'

'I think Muriel used to take us to school, but I mean it's only here. All you'd got to do is cross this road and another. Mind you, they was both busy roads. And then I remember going on my own a lot. I remember going on my own across here. I don't know how you felt, Sandra, but I didn't want Muriel to meet me. No way. I were a bit ashamed of her. I'm still like that. I was a nuisance at school. They were glad to get rid of me.'

'Used to get chased out of lessons, didn't you? "Not like your Sandra," they'd say.'

'I were just bad . . . bad influence on everybody. I think I had attitude, I've got an attitude problem. I got worse. . . . '

' . . . You're stronger than me. . . . '

' . . . when granddad died. I was eleven. I used to swear from little school. It was because Muriel used to take me out with all her friends at Doncaster and Rotherham. Because grandma never swore, granddad didn't. And I can't really remember Muriel swearing up till she became violent. . . . '

' . . . Yes, when she got violent she swore, but she didn't swear in general, did she?'

'I'd attitude up to about fourteen, when I, well up to about fourteen, fifteen when I had responsibilities of coming home and, you know, like looking after them. Grandma, she were full of arthritis.'

'She could still do though, she could still do.'

'Oh yes, she could still do things. But, I mean, grandma, she used to say she were dying . . . she were ill and she'd say, "I'm dying this time". That had a big effect on me. And I used to go to bed at night crying. If she's going to die, what's going to happen, you know. Big handful for grandma, Muriel was. I mean, like, when I took over, I sort of got, me and my grandma used to always argue because she'd give in to Muriel and I wouldn't.'

'I would, I'd give in to her.'

'They'd all give in to her, but I won't. Muriel'd say, "Buy me a packet of fags", she'd just smoked ten, I used to say, 'No. No. . . . '

'Grandma'd get her purse out, and Maggie and grandma'd be fighting, you know, arguing and not speaking then. . . . '

' . . . Because I wouldn't give in to her. She's a bugger for picking fags up off street now.'

'I mean she would ask you, even if you're smoking it, "Gives us that bit". And you know, it's . . . trying to tell people before you meet her.'

'Grandma did jobs. She did everything. She never really let Muriel do anything unless it was go and make a cup of tea . . . shopping, she'd go and fetch shopping.'

'Muriel would help with cleaning but she wouldn't do it properly, so grandma'd not bother. I learned Muriel, didn't I? I started to learn her. She'd do a bit of ironing. She'd only do one thing and say, "I've had enough now", and I'd say, "No, do it again". Then she'd do a bit more and it'd all be creased. I'd say, "No Muriel, that's not done properly, do it again". And I used to do it with Tracey, Tracey was the same. I mean, if it probably hadn't have been for me, Tracey'd have been worse than what she is. Like, sorting washing, grandma never showed them how, she used to just mollycoddle them. And then, same as washing pots, they'd wash pots and they'd be dirty. I'd say, "Do them again". And then she used to polish, I used to get Muriel to polish. I wasn't being, like, idle. It was just showing her what to do. But now she's gone to live with Bob, she doesn't do it. So all that's ruined. She knows, she knows how to do it. I don't know, I don't think Muriel'd be as bad as she is now. . . . I think grandma's done a lot. Mollycoddled her that much. Mind you, then again, grandma didn't probably have time with us three.'

'Yes, grandma'd give in for peace, wouldn't she?'

'It's only this last few years that I've been a bit better with Muriel. We've took her out. Me and boyfriend took her for her dinner on her birthday, and I thought, oh, I'm on edge. She's going to do summat, she's going to go walking across to somebody and say, "Hello, what's your name? Where do you come from?" And, like, she were eating that fast she went and choked and spit it out down her front. I said that's it, that's it, I shan't take her again. I was dead embarrassed.'

'She does put you on edge though, doesn't she? She's all right while she's all right, but then when she starts her calling, you know, I get so wound up. You know, start shouting, we start shouting and, you know.'

'She gets people just wound up dead quick. Dead quick, the way she mucks about . . . but I don't like anybody else calling her, especially people out of the family. That's my biggest thing, embarrassed, embarrassed of her.'

'Maggie's right. It's been like it all us lives. It was hard for me at school when they used to call her. There used to be a lot of people. . . .'

' . . . One-eyed jack. . . . '

' . . . yes, they used to call her like. But the friends I used to go about with, they all knew her, so they was all right with her. It was just the other children at school that used to call her. But, I mean, as for her never being married, that never cropped up. I can remember that never, ever come up.'

'I think, same as Sandra, if it's your close friends then you wouldn't mind so much. But if you'd met a new friend and, like, Muriel . . . I'd avoid her, I would avoid her.'

'She winds you up that much though, doesn't she? She winds us all, every one of us, everybody. I mean one particular time we had a solicitor's letter come to our house, and it said that I'd got to keep away – this was when grandma were alive – I'd got to keep away from this house, as when I come up I was begging money off her, I was begging money off her and I wouldn't leave her alone wanting money off her, isn't that right Maggie? Well, I come up here and I told my grandma. I mean we've never done it, never begged no money off her. We've always bought her fags. But that's it, that's where she is and then you have to accept her apology all time. She can do the evilest thing to you, and then it's, "Well, I'm sorry", you know. I mean she's had police, police to you, hasn't she Maggie?'

'Yes, no end of times.'

'Police have been down here, you know, and it's all a load of bull.'

'And then you're expected to forgive her. It's all, "I didn't mean anything I said." '

'It's you what have to forgive her.'

'And I say, "You've said it and that's it. I don't forgive you for it." I mean she's had some good hidings off our Anna's friend. She were that awful to grandma our Anna's best friend pinned her behind door and give her a good hiding, because she were that awful. But I always remember, I'd be about eight or nine, we'd got these great big dress-making scissors, she had them to my throat behind bathroom door. And I think granddad got hold of her over it. I don't know what I'd done wrong. And that's the only time. . . . '

' . . . She's never hit me. . . . '

' . . . and that's the only time I can remember her being violent to me. She's probably slapped us like normal, but she's never beat us. Never. Only them scissors I can remember, but I can't ever remember Muriel hitting us really. I remember she once hit grandma, the last time she hit grandma. This was when she was on needles. I was having nobody hit my grandma, nobody. I was about fourteen, fifteen, and I tell you, I hit her and knocked her straight over coffee table and split all her lip, and it upset me dead bad. I went crying down to my friend and I daren't tell her what I'd done. I mean we always say, you know, "Oh, Muriel, she's a nuisance, I hate her." But you don't really, not deep down.'

'I couldn't have her come and live with me. I couldn't cope with her. She'd send me to Middlewood, she would.'

'Nobody would, nobody'd have her.'

'Well, I'm always saying she's no mother to me. She never had been – has she? – never been a mother.'

'Grandma was our mother. She looked after us, grandma did. There was a time I can remember really as my first hug and that's when grandma died. Muriel put her arms round me and hugged me and I thought, I've never known her to do that. But now she'll come some-times. . . . '

' . . . She tends to do it a bit now, doesn't she? . . . '

' . . . if she's in a brilliant mood, she'll go round and kiss everybody. I mean first time she met Darryl, my boyfriend, she went and kissed him. I mean he says, "Oh, she's all right, leave her alone," but next time he met her she'd got it on, she had, and it shocked him. I says, "Darryl's never seen you like that", but she apologised for it.'

'There's Muriel here now! She is, Muriel's just come.'

'We're the same father, Maggie and me, but Tracey isn't. He's been about in the last year, two years.'

'Two year.'

'Two year ago. He's down Rotherham. I wouldn't know him if I passed him.'

'I would.'

'Yes, you would. I wouldn't.'

'Muriel found him out and we heard he was meeting her up Hanstead. Well, grandma's always brought us up, you know, grandma's always said don't want nothing to do with him. "He was never around when you was born," you know. When Muriel had Sandra he buggered off and then he come back, got her pregnant again, and he buggered off again. I says to our cousin Ellen, I says, would you know him? She says, "Yes." I says, come with me, I just want to have a look. We parked up Hanstead, and he was other side of market. Ellen said, "That's him!". I says, where? She says, "That's him, there!" I says, how can you tell from here? She says, "I'm telling you, that's him!". I was going to go and tell him to leave Muriel alone. I walked past him, walked past him again, crossed road, walked past him again, and this is all I could do. Just have a look. I thought, well, he looks fairly clean, he looks all right. He looked quite smart. And I never went up to him.'

'Grandma always told us that he stood up in court and said we wasn't his, didn't he Maggie? That's as much as we know.'

'She never had a penny from him, grandma, and she never had nothing from anybody.'

'He just said they're not mine and that's that. That's all we've been brought up to him saying, that we're not his, so. . . .'

'We've met Tracey's father.'

'Well, I've never met him.'

'I have. Muriel brought him home. I remember he sat me on his knee and I didn't like him. He was Italian. Mario. Mario were his name and I didn't like him. I know I didn't want to go with them. If Muriel'd got a house anywhere I wouldn't have gone, and you wouldn't, would you Sandra?'

'No.'

'I'd have stopped with grandma.'

'Muriel was only saying this week she'd just had a letter from our dad. He's been in contact with her again. I wouldn't read it though.'

'It's only this last couple of years since grandma died. . . . '

'Yes, that she's been in contact.'

'She'll find him out. Samaritans she'll go to. She'll find anybody out, Muriel would. We've always been brought up never to have nothing to do with him. Haven't we?'

'Yes. I've never really wanted. I'm not interested.'

'I probably would've wanted to have known him if it hadn't been for grandma.'

'Grandma used to get help from social services and health authorities, things like that. She'd go so long and then she needed a break. And then they'd send Muriel to Bank House for a fortnight. That's about it really. I think this was when you'd left Sandra, wasn't it? . . . '

' . . . It would be. . . . '

' . . . when they started to help with things like that, when grandma got older and she couldn't cope. She used to go for weekend here, to give grandma a break, weekend there, you know, or a fortnight away, which did give us all a break. It were like a cloud had lifted when she'd gone. You know, everything'd be nice, there'd be no falling out or anything. There was always an atmosphere because of Muriel. Oh, and Tracey went out fostered a couple of times. I remember that was hard.'

'When was it when she went to that woman at Bessacarr, Maggie? How old was she then?'

'Thirteen, fourteen. And then she went to a woman down Blaxton and I'd got friends from school there and I had to take her down, not Muriel or grandma. I had to take our Tracey down and show her everywhere and there were like two lads from our school that had got no parents and she'd adopted them. Oh God, I remember that, that was horrible. And I went up to them at school and I had to say, "Please don't tell anybody". That was really dead bad. To think that my sister had got to be fostered out. Because I don't think they knew about Muriel, there was only a few people that knew about Muriel at big school. You know, like, when you're a teenager you've got attitude problem and everything. Every time you got new friends you'd have to start over again. Like, if you're bringing them home, then you would have to explain, and it's horrible. I'd just say my mum's. . . . '

' . . . Not right. . . . '

' . . . No, I'd say she's a bit backward. And then I'd have to go through it and say well, when grandma were, when she was carrying Muriel she got double pneumonia and it. . . . '

' . . . Had she? . . . '

' . . . caused Muriel to be backward. The doctor told grandma don't buy all these things because there may not be any baby. That's what I've always had to explain to people. I've had to go right through it, so I wouldn't feel so bad. I wouldn't, like, say, well, Muriel's backward. I'd have to go all the way through it to blame double pneumonia for it. I'd say you just have to be careful with her, you know, and she'll come up to you and all these questions she'll say to people. Just have to warn them like that, it's horrible.'

'I don't even know what actually to say about her, what she is.'

'They can't class her as mentally handicapped. Or like backward. They class her as learning difficulties. It doesn't sound so bad. There's nothing to put her in, they can't put her in any class.'

'My main friends, I more or less had them all from junior school like all the way through to big school.'

'It was our Anna that used to say if they can't accept her then that's their problem, they're no friend. And I've always stuck by what our Anna said. I thought if they wouldn't accept her or take mickey, then I wouldn't be close to them. There's some people at work – isn't there, Sandra? – and I think well, I'm not telling them.'

'Maggie wouldn't tell them. I would. I'd tell them what she's like. You never know where Muriel's going to turn up, so I try and explain best I can how she is.'

'They probably know anyway.'

'We do worry because one of girls at work, she did see her down Bawtry. She says, "Oh, I know who your mum is now," and I'd go bright red. I thought oh, did she pick up a fag or was she talking to herself, because she talks to herself an all, you know.'

'And yet I'm more closer to Muriel – aren't I? – than you, and I'm the one that daren't tell people. It hurts, I don't know, it just does. Muriel's who she is, I should accept that. But, like, well, it was at your wedding, Sandra, and she was acting a bit silly, and I said if I ever get married she's not being there. Because of all my friends. I'd be on edge all day.'

'Well, we was. We was on edge. I said to Maggie, like, we said, "Watch her, Maggie. Make sure, you know, she's right".'

'But I was on edge all day having to watch her.'

'Well, we were all on edge. I said, I'm telling you, Muriel, if you start messing about, you're going. We do aggravate her. But when she's in the right mood, we can have a laugh with her.'

'I wouldn't do that at one time, I wouldn't be seen out with her. It were only since grandma died and then, like, we take her walks, we took her out for a meal. Where did we take her, Sandra, somewhere like Alton Towers?'

'Yes, we took her there. We're always threatening her though. As we're walking along we can be saying, "I'm telling you, you don't speak to nobody that you shouldn't do", you know. Because she would talk to people . . . or we're frightened of her asking them for a fag or . . . picking one up.'

'I think if I ever took her shopping, and I've got friends at Bawtry, you see, where I work, I'd never take her there. Even though I've told a few people about her.'

' . . . She does, she puts you all on edge.'

'We've got a wedding coming up in September, haven't we Sandra? I shall be all on edge there because they'll not be just family there. . . . '

' . . . But she's not missed out, they'll not miss her out because of it.'

'Well, if we didn't want to go to school we didn't have to go, did we Maggie? Grandma'd say, "Don't go today, I'm not very well", and we didn't used to go.'

'I was always having school bobby. Like Sandra says, grandma would say, "Don't go to school, I'm not very well today". So week after, I'd think, well, I'm not very well so I'm not going. You see, I was ever so crafty, always having school bobby. They once come up stairs and fetched me. I hated school, hated it. I thought it were a drag, couldn't wait to leave.'

'I liked both the two little schools, but when it come to going to big school, I didn't like that. I'd never wish like some people that I were back at school. I hated it. I've always been one to pull myself down. I think I can't do it before I've even had a go. If it's putting pen to paper, I can't do it, but if it's anything to do with my hands I'll have a go. At school, I was dreading having to read or anything like that in front of class. I liked PE, running. At junior school I won everything. I got a little trophy for that, nobody could beat me. And when I got into big school I used to like PE and maths, but that was the only two. Oh, and community service – when you go out to old people and nursery schools and things like that.'

'I was a good runner at Maltby Road, same as Sandra. I won everything. I think that come from granddad – didn't it? – because he was a runner, he was a runner for district. I liked cooking towards the end, like in the fourth and fifth years, but everything else, it was boring. Couldn't be bothered with it. Only thing I was good in at school was community service when I used to have to go out and look after old people, go and clean their windows, and they always used to praise me for that. Couldn't do it for a job, it'd upset me too much. I'd love it, but I'd, like, get dead close to them – wouldn't I? – and it'd upset me. I mean I'm hard in some ways, but I'm a softie, I'm ever so soft. Owt can make me cry.'

'Yet you could stand up for yourself to anybody.'

'I tell anybody what I think of them. But soft really.'

'I left school at fifteen and I worked straight away then. I met Andrew when I were seventeen at a darts' match, when I'd just started going out. I went into hosiery, I was on a machine, and then I left to have William. And then only other job I've had since then has been Fox's. We work machines there, don't we Maggie?'

'I were working before I left school. I used to make, like, little tiles for front of fireplaces. Then they finished me there and I went doing plastics, spot welding, a glass-making job. Give me a drill, hammer and nails, I'm right. You give me a sewing needle I don't know what to do. . . . '

' . . . She could do a bloke's job. . . . '

' . . . and then I got evening job at Fox's, didn't I, and ever since I've been stuck there.'

'We've always seemed to work, haven't we Maggie? In fact, we're probably most that's worked in the family.'

'Yes. Harder it is the more I like it. I love hard work, love it.'

'Them next door, she's got three girls and they're all older than us and I can't honestly say they've ever worked much at all in their lives. It's Muriel's older sister next door. Their daughter next door to that, there's three in a row.'

'Somebody asked me at work, they said, "God, how big's your family?" I says I don't really know, and I got to 105. There's between twenty-five and thirty of us in family that's all dead close. We see each other every week. I mean, we call each other but you guarantee if anything goes wrong, we're there, we all stick together.'

'Grandma had three daughters, Muriel, Marion and Anna. Muriel had three daughters, Marion had three daughters and a son, and our Anna's had a son and daughter. There seem to be more girls in family than boys. Even with lads, they're still quite close.'

'All my friends now are at Fox's, I've not got no other friends.

Because, like, when I was about fifteen, when I did take over at home and I were working, I didn't have time. I lost all my friends with looking after grandma. I never used to go out. But I say if I had my time to go back, I'd do it all again, do it all again. She looked after us, grandma did. So my friends are all at Fox's. And I just didn't want to leave there when grandma died. I mean I could've thought well, I'll go and get a day job now. But I like it there.'

'And I've got all older friends. I stick with older friends, I do, a lot older. I do prefer older company. Better than younger ones. I don't know why. . . . '

' . . . Because of grandma. And I'm more family, aren't I Sandra? I stick with family, it's just me.'

'But you caused me some trouble as I got to sixteen, as I left school. You was a sod, you know Maggie.'

'I think I was just unhappy because of Muriel . . . because I hadn't got a dad, my mum. . . . '

'That's never bothered me.'

' . . . wasn't right. Eh?'

'That's never bothered me.'

'It has me. It has me. Like, Muriel wasn't right. I think it's done a big effect on my life, Muriel being as she is. I'm always scared of what other people are thinking, and I've always thought people are better than me, always. You couldn't bring people home like a normal family. And, you know with families now, it'll upset me if I go to somebody's house and they're shouting and arguing. It'll upset me dead bad and I won't go, I hate that. But I mean like clothes. I always had your hand-me-downs, didn't I Sandra?'

'I had secondhand.'

'Yes, but you had more than me, Sandra. I mean I had all your hand-me-downs. But then Tracey had more than us, more than all of us.'

'Yes, we struggled. Till more or less after my granddad died and my grandma had all money. It seemed to pick up then because my gran was claiming money for Muriel, for our Tracey, you know, and she seemed to get plenty then.'

'I were terrible I was. I used to be a right dirty mouth, swearing terrible. It'd be lads I'd be fighting with, not girls, lads. It's from when I were little. Mainly, I reckon, because I was with Muriel more. She used to take me out.'

'When you used to want to come with me I used to go running up street. I wouldn't take her. I always used to be frightened of Maggie. She used to belt me, she did. And she'd hit you with anything, anything she could pick up. I had to run and lock the door so she couldn't get at me. Violent, like Muriel, she was. She was nasty.'

'And I'm ashamed of it. I'm ashamed, the things I've done. Awful. I know what I was when I were a kid. And I've always said, if I'd been grandma I'd have had me put away. I would. I would have had me put away. Because I were that bad. Our Tracey was very unruly an' all. She were fostered twice. She used to throw tantrums like Muriel. With grandma being old and Muriel being as she is, well I think they could have done with a bit more help.'

'I don't think we got any, did they? It were just lecturing.'

'Yes, it was just lecturing. They just used to talk and not really do anything. Well, they didn't lecture Tracey all that much. She was very unruly. She got worse as teenager – didn't she, Sandra? – up to when she left school and started work. We got her on at our place, packing. She were only there up to Christmas and she was as right as rain, no problems, and then she got laid off. Then it started, didn't it? She used to go to Bessacarr because she'd got nowt to do. Different friends and stopping out all night, and I wouldn't have it. I was very protective, you know, because that's when grandma had died. I thought, "Oh God, if she comes home pregnant." I used to say you've got to help in the house, but she didn't like it. I got on to her that much about helping. I used to say you're not using it as a hotel, I'll kick you out, but I didn't mean it. When I were at work one day, she come with boyfriend, took all her stuff. I didn't know where she'd gone. She'd been gone for months, hadn't she Sandra? I was going crazy. I was hunting round Bessacarr. You'd seen her up Kenwell. We were chasing them round in car. Then I think Muriel left a message at dole office saying could Tracey Lewis contact her family. And she did, you see.'

'She's twenty-one next month but she is difficult, she is. She's a lot like Muriel, a lot like her.'

'She's sensible, isn't she, sometimes. She'll be as good as gold and then all of a sudden she'll create and you'll see her get all high and start acting silly, won't she Sandra? Her boyfriend's back now. He went in prison. We think he was driving and he'd been banned and he'd no MOT or anything. Baby got meningitis when he was in prison. That did me, didn't it?'

'Only a few month ago it were, in April. Baby was just eleven month old. That upset us, didn't it?'

'Baby were ever so badly and they kept saying she's got flu. I knew, I knew how she was holding her head. Doctor come and they rushed her in. I just walked out crying. I were at hospital all that night with her, laid in my arms, baby was. She's to go for tests to see if it's affected anything like her liver or kidneys and hearing and everything else. She's still going through all them, but she seems all right, doesn't she Sandra?'

'They always say I went off rails when granddad died. Isn't that right, Sandra? I had my hair shaved down sides. I pierced my nose myself. I had my hair all colours there was, didn't I? I used to be punk rocker – studs round neck, studs all here, studs all on my jacket. Smoking. Fighting. Pinching. I did do a lot of pinching. But now, I wouldn't do anybody out of penny, you know, I would never sleep. I think I were leader. I used to go out with a lad, he were a punk rocker, and he used to be like me. His parents had split up and he'd been kicked out house. I bought a motorbike. Grandma wouldn't agree to that, but I bought it. I'd be fourteen, fifteen. I had a big 125 motorbike. Couldn't even touch floor with it, but I bought it just to be big. Anything to be big. Mick Turbot learnt me to pinch. He used to go up to shop up here and he'd say, you ask for a bottle of milk. She used to go round back for bottle of milk while he used to nick chocolate off of front. I got done for that. Police come and give me a right telling off. Then I used to muck about with our Sheila – that's when I started smoking and pinching and fighting. She was a big influence on me, Sheila was. I remember a lot of people wouldn't let their kids play with me. Stamfords, you know, they wouldn't, and Pauline up here, her mam and dad didn't want her going with me. But I think now, I mean Stamfords, he's been in nick and all lot, and I think to myself, well, I've turned out a hell of a lot better than a lot of them.'

'I wouldn't dare do anything like that. I can always remember a girl that were same age as me, she lived up at pub at top of road. She used to pinch out of till and give it to me. We used to go down onto rec and, like, get drink and chocolates and we'd be smoking down there. I think once our Anna caught me and belted me. I never had another go. But I was sort of always the wimpy one, daren't do it myself. At work now, like, I'll say Maggie, you do this, and she'll do it because I daren't. Then we both crack up laughing. We have some, ever such fun. But I daren't do it. I'm all for easy life. With any arguing or anything like that, I just try and calm it down.'

'Where I'll go in straight.'

'I've got to be really, really wound up before I explode.'

'You let people walk all over you. And I've had that. People's walked over me and I won't have it any more. I don't like people taking advantage of me. Detention and lines we had at school. Once when I had my hair shaved I had to stop outside headmistress' class. She wouldn't let me go back in class with my hair like it was, it had to grow back. So I just sat outside office all time. When teachers had gone out, we'd go in and nick jotters, books and things like that. So that did no good. Grandma used to say, "Right, you can stop in". No way would I, I'd be out.'

'I can't remember being punished. If anybody punished us it'd have been our Anna.'

'I've had board rubbers chucked at me by teacher, I'd wind her up that much. She locked me in class and I were climbing out window and she caught me.'

'Teachers always used to say to you, "You're not like your Sandra".'

'I once got suspended. We'd been drinking. It was nearly Christmas time and there was one of these parties for fifth years. We all went home at dinner and went back drunk. Well, I don't think we were drunk, probably about ten of us shared a bottle of cider. We all started chucking these miniature sausages all round, and one hit Mr Dunwoody. They checked me and sent my fags and lighter home. Grandma never knew I smoked till then.'

'Biggest effect in my life was when grandma died. That is the biggest thing. Muriel lived here a year after grandma died. I felt awful when she left. I thought, God, I bet everybody thinks I've kicked her out now. But it was Muriel what wanted to go. I mean, I have been bad with her, Sandra, haven't I? She's wound me up sometimes dead bad.'

'We swear, don't we?'

'Well, you don't swear all that much. I mean you feel more resentful against her, don't you, than me? I used to say I hate her guts, I hate her. But then I thought to myself, probably something had happened, like probably when I hit her that time, and I thought no, you don't hate her. And I don't really say it now Sandra, do I?'

'No.'

'I used to say it all the time, I hate you, you're not my mother. She was quite good when grandma died. I mean I bottle it all up and I think Muriel does as well. I think she was more over granddad, wasn't she? She used to go down and lie on his grave. People used to come to me and say your Muriel were lying on your granddad's grave crying. I really wasn't all old enough to help her through it. When grandma died, I were that bad, wasn't I Sandra? Always crying and things like that. I blamed Muriel and Tracey at first. I used to say grandma'd still been here now if it hadn't been for you two, what you've put grandma through, you've killed her. And that must have hurt them rotten. I blamed everybody, didn't I? I took it out on my best friends, took it out on everybody, I did. I couldn't handle it. She come home Monday night and she died Tuesday morning. She'd got up and she'd opened her curtains. Grandma always used to say, "I can't wait for daylight". I think she was frightened of dying at night.'

'I couldn't believe it. Our Anna rang me up and said grandma'd died and I put phone down. I had to ring her back and see, you know, if it was. . . . '

'I remember our Anna phoning me up and I just didn't take it in. Because she says oh, we can't wake my mam up. So she says will you go round and tell Marion. Well, I thought to myself, stupid idiot, she'll be all right when I get over there, he'll have woke her up. Well anyway, everybody started gathering here and I were just whistling, I were hoovering round happy. I wouldn't take it. And they says just go and look at her. . . . '

'You were screaming though. I said leave her, leave her.'

'I wouldn't let her go, I just held her. I didn't handle it very good. I never want to go through that again. I think it's only since last year I'm all right again, I'm back to normal. Took me a hell of a long time. Great lady. Grandma was the best.'

'The only time I remember Muriel putting her arms round me was at the funeral. I remember grandma used to hug me. I used to sit with grandma and put my arms round her when I were little. I've learnt to be that bit more loving, where Sandra won't, will you?'

'No.'

'Learnt it from our Anna and her kids. From seeing her with her kids. I mean I'm always getting hold of kids, aren't I?'

'I don't with William. I mean I did when he were little.'

'Yes, but you've put that onto him now, haven't you? I mean I would, I'd go up to him and hug him and kiss him.'

'Yes, but he'd say get off.'

'Yes, he wouldn't have it. Our Sam, how old's our Sam? Twelve. He'll come and give me a kiss. I don't think it's right to be like we are. I mean our Ellen nearly lost her husband, she was crying. There was me, her two sisters, her dad and mam, and not one went to comfort her and it upset me. I'll never forget it. I think it's wrong. She was crying other week because her sister were rushed in hospital and I thought to myself, it's not going to happen again, so I went to put my arm round her. So I've learnt that bit more now, where I wouldn't have done before. Our

Marion is same, she can't go and hug her own daughters. But our Anna's different. She's brought them up to show their feelings, but we haven't. I'm always mucking about with kids but I don't want none myself. No way. All trouble they cause.'

'All worry they cause.'

'Yes. I'm more animals. Don't know why. I'm terrible – aren't I? – the way I feel for them. Like she feels for William, I'm there with animals. I think because I'd got nobody to love, I've clung to them. I mean you've got Andrew and William, but I've clung to animals. You don't want any more kids, do you Sandra?'

'No, I've just never wanted no more. Andrew says he'd like a little girl. Well, it's tough. I think I wouldn't, not now, at my age and William being that age. I don't think I've got patience as well with them.'

'I think it's important to show love.'

'I feel as though I've got none to show. For nobody. Maggie always says I only love myself and love William.'

'I'll go to Sandra and say, I loves you, Sandra, she'll say, "Oh, get lost." It's weird. I mean we must have had love, but we was never . . . I don't know . . . we wasn't, like, hugged all the time. It was probably only when we went to grandma. It's somewhere from a long time ago that's gone wrong, and it's passed on to all us. Not so much me now. I don't think it's right. I just don't think it's right. Like when grandma were in hospital, you never went to kiss her, did you Sandra? I used to go and kiss her. Or, like, our Marion's birthday, I mean she's old and I kissed her. I think I did it for first time this year. She was probably a bit shocked.'

'I think I could do with somebody to talk to. I bottle things up.'

'She's terrible, terrible. I've learnt her a bit.'

'Mmm. . . . '

' . . . I mean you tell me some things, don't you? You should be able to talk to each other. It's all wrong. I just bottle it up and try and sort it out myself. So she's not like on her own there, we're the same for that. We can't talk to each other. I don't trust people, that's my problem. I don't trust people and I wouldn't tell, if I'd got a problem, you know.'

'We've never had a decent present off Muriel, have we? I mean some-times at Christmas Sandra'd get more and I wouldn't get nowt hardly. Even now I might not come off with owt and she might get a present.'

'I mean you never get nothing really decent off her, like any other parent, like I do with William. He gets something good for birthdays, everything. She's got no idea, no idea at all. You get nothing. I think only thing I've ever had, when I got married I got that Lilliput Lane Cottage. You know, but she's no idea how to buy for anybody.'

'Even like when we were young, I remember her getting me summat like 50p book. I used to think God, every other kid gets loads and I get 50p off her. And I bet you I'd probably chuck it at her. If I were like twelve, I'd say you can stuff it, I don't want it, I would. Grandma used to give her £25 and it went on nothing. This is why you have to watch her. You can give her £100, she'll go and waste it, and she'll come back to you saying, "Can I have some fags?" No matter what you give her, she'll still come back. But sometimes she'll come down with some biscuits for dog, "Here you are, I've bought you these." I'll say, you shouldn't do it, Muriel, it's your money, go and buy something for yourself. But heart's there, you know.'

'I feel . . . I don't feel as though I've got . . . I mean, I feel as though I've got no love for her. If anything happened to her, I think that'd be different again. I feel I've got no love for her, I haven't. I mean, I don't know, just makes me feel sick. She sent me a birthday card – it were my birthday other day – and it were just a plain birthday card, happy birthday on it. But somebody else had wrote in it, just "To Sandra from Mum." You know, not even one with "Daughter" on. But no, I wouldn't say I've got any love for her at all. I feel as though she thought less for me than any of others. Muriel didn't have much at all to do with me. Even now I'd say I was the less thought of. Even though she rang me up on my birthday, you know, and there were just her and my friend that rang me up, like, on my birthday. But I do think I'm last. It does hurt. I thought, I'll just wait till Maggie's birthday and see if she gets a card with "Daughter" on.'

'I used to say I hated her. I mean I used to feel like you till I hit her and made her mouth bleed and it upset me, and I think then I realised I must have feelings for her. If anybody harmed her, I'd kill them. I mean I could say oh God, she gets on my nerves, I hate her guts. But I've looked into it more than that. I've a lot of feelings for her. I think you have got feelings for her if anything happened to her, Sandra. I know you.'

'Yes, that's what I'm saying. I'd probably be different again if something happened. I wouldn't want her not here. No, I wouldn't want her not here, no.'

'Although she's a nuisance, she's created heartache and everything, it'd be horrible without her.'

'In fact I think our Tracey, younger one, now is quite cruel to her, isn't she Maggie? She seems to be. Muriel says that she went down last

week and Tracey told her to get off and shouting after her get off. I
mean, I wouldn't do that if she come to my house. I'd have her in and
say, don't touch that, because she's into everything. You're following her,
when she comes. It's not that she comes to our house much, once in a
blue moon, but I'm all on edge. Muriel is what she is, you know. I can
only take so much of her and I could just scream at her.'

'She comes here two and three times a week, probably more. She
used to come on a Sunday night and stop for a few hours, but since I've
been courting we're probably going out on a Sunday night.'

'I see her here. She mostly comes here every Friday, doesn't she
Maggie? And she doesn't stop very long. I mean we've had a laugh with
her – haven't we? – have a laugh and joke with her. We'd go a walk and
she's right as rain then. It's just when she starts, I can't be doing with it.
I just don't want it.'

'I mean I've turned her away many a time. She come yesterday, she
could drop in anytime.'

'We don't really visit her, not really. I never actually go, have a cup of
tea there or anything like that. I see her here.'

'It's always here. She's had her name down for a house since we were
little.'

'They won't give her one.'

'They keep trying to train her up but nobody'll have her. I mean
when she lived here, I thought oh God, I can't stand it. But now she's
gone I feel sorry, and I feel guilty that she's gone out of her own home
that she's been brought up in and I've got it – but I didn't push her out,
she wanted to go. But I still feel guilty. I know what grandma felt about
Muriel. She used to say, "Never have her put away", didn't she Sandra?
Never, never have her put away. And that's stuck with me you see. I
wouldn't.'

'But where does she belong? I mean, I think whoever looks after her
wants a thousand pound a week. Because she's terrible, she is terrible.
She comes down here, shout, moaning about that. I mean we're all
right one minute just talking, then she'll go on about something else,
calling them black and blue. And then she's swearing about them and
all things like that. And you lose your patience then, you don't want her.
You want her gone, straight away.'

'Our Alice were saying other day she'd gone past training centre
where Muriel is. She were standing there waiting for bus and all of
them round her were like pulling their pants up, like shouting, and she
thought, "Oh, Muriel doesn't belong there at all".'

'Yes. There's a lot of Down's syndromes or what have you there, isn't there?'

'It sort of like touched me when she told me. And I just sat there thinking, you know, she shouldn't be with them sort of people. They said it's like a training place. I mean we didn't say we want her putting there, it was them that come to us. It was them that decided, like, to get her out of the way of grandma you see. Because grandma wasn't all that young so it used to get Muriel out. But I mean I've been quite a few times. I mean she's a nuisance, yes, but I bet she's the only one there that's right in head, you know, properly. It can't be nice for her.'

'I don't think she could manage. . . . '

'Grandma mollycoddled her. Always done for her. And we've not . . . and all family's not helped. She'd have been a different person. She might have been that bit backward, but she wouldn't have been as bad. That's what makes me mad. She can do it. If somebody learned her to look after her money. . . . There was all big plans at training place, "We'll get her to do this, we'll get her to do that". They've ruined her, they've ruined her as well, doing everything for her. Responsibility's all gone now, you see. She's got very bad . . . a lot of bad points, but, like, if you ask her for help then she'll help you. Not so long ago I had a lot of trouble with my back – didn't I Sandra? – and I couldn't go to work. I says to Muriel, will you come down for week and look after me? She was as good as gold, she couldn't do enough. And I'd do it again, if I wasn't very well, I'd ask her, wouldn't I? I'd say will you come down, and she'd love it.'

'She looked after you more than she did me. She didn't really have a lot to do with me, did she?'

'No, I wouldn't say looked after, I mean she took me out with her and things like that. But cooking, all things like that, washing and ironing I used to do all of that. She always took us to doctor's.'

'Yes. Anything wrong with you . . . she always took us to things like that more than grandma. I will say that.'

'And you always remember, like you didn't want Muriel, when you were badly, you always cried grandma. I've put myself in Muriel's place sometimes, because I would, I would see it as rejection.'

'But I've always felt as though, whatever you say to her, she just lets it go in there and straight out other end.'

'Yes, but she's got to have feelings, hasn't she? She'll have feelings like the rest of us. I know sometimes you think it goes in and out. . . . '

' . . . Well, we've not treated her right.'

'Well, we haven't, because we've not been treated right. You can't say she was a mother.'

'No, I didn't. But I just think you can say what you want to her and it wouldn't bother her. It wouldn't upset her like it would me.'

'But that poinsettia I got on Sunday. I told her off Sunday. I went crazy at her and she's gone and brought me that. Now if it goes in one ear and out other, she wouldn't have bothered. But it must have played on her mind to come back and bought that.'

'Sandra knows. This house means a lot to me. I don't want to move.'

'I always said you wouldn't.'

'No, it means a lot to me this house, where I grew up and grandma's house, something she cherished. I don't think people realise.'

'Yes, it means a lot to everybody. We've always lived here, always.'

'I live in dreams. I used to think I wished I'd got a mam and dad . . . wished I'd got, you know, parents. . . . '

'I can never remember being unhappy.'

' . . . But then again, if Muriel'd, you know, if she'd been a proper mum, I think, well, we wouldn't have probably had grandma so much, I wouldn't have been so close to grandma so. . . . What do you think, Sandra?'

'I'd say we were happy enough. Would you? Well, I was.'

POSTSCRIPT

I would just like to say and make sure it gets across that although Muriel is difficult and no matter what she has done and how much trouble she causes I will never have her put away in care. Also she will always be loved by all the family just the same. I would like to ask a special favour if I could I would like to dedicate my part of the book to my grandma for looking after my mother and for raising me in such a special way and if you could leave her name the same which is Mary Ann. Yours faithfully, M. Lewis.

Chapter 7

Two lives revisited

Sometimes people's stories are so compelling that as researchers we are best letting them speak for themselves. Bogdan and Taylor (1976) long ago urged us to reflect less and listen more as an aid to understanding. We have followed their example in recounting Maggie and Sandra's story in the previous chapter.

However, the standing of such an unadorned account of personal experience remains a matter of dispute. In one camp are those who argue the importance of readers engaging directly with the story rather than with the author who produced the text. The strength of narrative lies precisely in its capacity to draw readers into the 'worlds created in the words' (Scheppele, 1989) through the power of the imagination. Allowing an authorial voice to intrude detracts from both the dramatic force of the story and its authenticity. From this point of view, 'unelaborated concreteness' (Abrams, 1991) – a concentration on the details of the story without resort to abstraction – is more true to the experience it seeks to portray. Ownership of the story too rests where it lies instead of being countermanded by the researcher's claim to interpret its significance.

On the other side of the narrative divide are those, like Clandinin and Connelly (1994), who maintain that 'researchers cannot stop there'. Stories must move beyond the concrete and the particular if they are to advance our understanding. They must be shown to have meaning to others beyond their teller. This calls for analysis in order to draw out their generic characteristics and the narrative threads that connect them to other lives. It is hard to dispute a straightforward account of personal experience. By contrast, it is possible to assess the validity or persuasiveness of the argument that a personal narrative contains features that make it also the story of a group. Only when stories are rounded off by analysis can they be said to constitute scholarship as opposed to mere anecdote.

We are torn between these two points of view and persuaded by each in turn. On the one hand, we are wary of the dangers inherent in the research relationship of misappropriating other people's experience for selfish ends. On the other hand, as researchers, we do not accept that silence is the only permissible response to the stories people tell. The forms of the previous chapter and this one reflect this position. In the last chapter, the sisters, Sandra and Maggie, were allowed to speak for themselves. In this chapter we use their story as raw material for analysis.

Peacock and Holland (1993) identify two approaches to the use of life stories in the social sciences: one which emphasises the 'life' while the other emphasises the 'story'. The life-focused approach is concerned primarily with the dynamics of lives as providing a window on the world of events and experience. The story-focused approach is concerned primarily with the dynamics of narration and the process by which lives are turned into text. Runyan (1984) makes a similar distinction between life stories as 'lives in the world' and as 'accounts of lives'. In each case the point is the same: narrative is both 'phenomenon and method' (Connelly and Clandinin, 1990). It constitutes a topic of study as well as a method of enquiry. In this chapter, we examine the sisters' tale from both these angles.

NARRATIVE AS STRUCTURED EXPERIENCE

Why pick on Maggie and Sandra? What can we hope to learn from their experience of growing up? These questions go to the heart of the narrative method. For critics, any one story stands alone, waiting to be contradicted by the next person who comes along with a different tale to tell. One life provides no basis for talking about all lives. For the prophets of narrative this criticism misses the point. Narrative should not be judged against criteria devised for other forms of research. Its purpose is not generalisation but 'transferability'. The test is whether there are elements of this particular story that may be treated as what Thomas and Znaniecki (1958) called 'mere instances' of a more general narrative and as such help to illuminate human experience.

Most people would hesitate to name a social scientist who had contributed more than Shakespeare to our understanding of the human condition. The same goes for most great dramatists and novelists. Their achievements are not realised by working from the particular to the general but by embodying the general in the particular. Their tools are the dramatic qualities of character, plot, scene, event and action rather than the rules of evidence. Human experience shows the same sort of storied qualities. People organise their memory largely in the form of narrative. But the stories people tell about their lives and their mode of telling are not solely of their own making. They also show the stamp of the wider communities to which they belong. By 'listening beyond' the particularities of their individual story it is possible to pick up the narrative threads that connect them to others who share their experience. Just as the artist 'searches for the universal in the one' (Sandelowski, 1994) so also do the singular, concrete details of people's lives achieve what Bruner (1991) calls an 'emblematic status' as part of a story that is in some sense generic.

George Eliot gives us another reason for attending to a single story in all its uniqueness. Analysis based on generalisations and statistics, she argued, calls for 'a sympathy ready-made, a moral sentiment already in activity'. A feeling for the subject is required in order to render such abstractions meaningful. The great function of the novelist was, for her, 'the extension of our sympathies'. She saw her role as that of an 'imaginative historian, even scientific investigator' (Ashton, 1994) whose method was to analyse political and social change through human stories in such a way that an individual's destiny is seen to be shaped by these historical changes as they happen. The great purpose of her storytelling – and, she believed, of all art – was to convey a picture of human life that would compel readers to pay attention 'to what is apart from themselves' and so 'extend our contact with our fellow-men beyond the bounds of our personal lot' (Eliot, 1963). Such a sentiment encapsulates the lure of the narrative method. Narrative research is about using personal stories to amplify our experience. We know next to nothing about the lives of children whose parents have learning difficulties nor about what it means to be a child in such a family. Yet social workers, psychologists, teachers, nurses, educationalists, judges and others who exercise the power to intervene in their lives are often required to make judgements about what is in their best interests which presume just such an understanding. The only way for them to fill the void is to project themselves into the child's position. Such attempts at empathy come at a price. They often mean that children's experience is filtered through the values of mainly middle-class professionals and assessed against standards that have no place in their world. This is why it is important to listen at length to the likes of Maggie and Sandra. Their story, as George Eliot would have it, widens our sympathies by enabling us to engage with their lives at the level of feeling as well as knowing.

The language of science does not easily accommodate the emotional dimension of human experience. Indeed, scientific discourse tends rather to treat human emotions as contaminants that threaten to compromise the ideal of objectivity. This point goes to the heart of what passes for knowledge about other people's lives. Sandelowski (1994) makes plain the distinction between propositional and universal truths. Propositional truths are truths *about* the world. Universal truths are about being true *to* life. Science is typically concerned with the former where art strives to embrace the latter. The language of science may be a perfect medium for discovering truths about a world of facts, but it cannot express life which is about more than mere facts. We need a poetic of inquiry that encompasses the realm of feelings in order to render human experience intelligible. This is the contribution of narrative which seeks precisely to bridge the gap between a literal and a figurative conception of reality. The story of the two sisters provides a test of this claim.

Having provided a justification for focusing on just one story let us now move on to examine the features that make it also the story of a group.

The importance of family

Maggie and Sandra were lucky growing up, as they did, in a large, tightly knit family. Maggie once got to 105 before she stopped counting her relatives. Twenty-five to thirty of them are 'all dead close': seeing each other every week, sharing anniversaries, partying together ('We've always had, like, parties . . . you know, all girls'll get together and we'll all, cakes and things, we always do that'), sticking up for each other in times of trouble ('I mean we call each other, but anything goes wrong we're there'). As many as ten all go biking together at weekends. Sharing and togetherness were part of Maggie and Sandra's upbringing ('We were never left out, was we?'), crammed as they were into their grandparents' semi with their mother and an aunt, Muriel's younger sister. It was 'granddad for bills' and grandma for most else. Their Aunt Anna used to keep them in order, disciplining them with a firm hand ('She used to belt us, didn't she?'). Maggie now says, 'I respect her for that.' She 'looked up' to her aunt, hoping that she'd grow up 'dead pretty' like her. Another aunt, their mother's elder sister, lived next door. She had four children, all older than Maggie and Sandra, one of whom, a daughter, now lives two doors away. As Sandra says, 'there's three in a row'. When Sandra upped and left home at eighteen she went to stay with one of her many cousins. There was always someone to turn to when the need arose. Throughout their childhood the family has been a safe haven. 'I stick with family,' said Maggie. Quite apart from the security and comfort and practical assistance it offers, the family is important for its unconditional acceptance of Muriel as a person. With outsiders, 'you're always having to warn people'. There is no need to explain or apologise for her to relatives. Even though 'she's done summat horrible to everybody', nobody (and 'there's a lot of us') 'really misses her out'. Children in the study who lacked the sound anchorage provided by Maggie and Sandra's family generally took more of a pounding.

The family in the community

Three generations had passed through Maggie and Sandra's family home. It has been in the family for over sixty years. Maggie has no wish to move; her sister always said she wouldn't. 'It means a lot to me this house,' Maggie says. 'It means a lot to everyone,' Sandra adds.

Their street was 'one of the best'; the 'neighbours were brilliant'. Everyone knew each other, 'even right to top of street'. The kids all played together, there were street parties, and a street collection when-ever anyone died, usually organised by grandma. Maggie recalls how Nancy next door used to send round bowls of chips, 'because she knew we used to have to struggle'. Sandra often spent the day with her instead of going to school. Jack and Peggy the other side were the same. The street's 'gone downhill' a bit in recent years. There's not many of the old families left, or so Maggie says until they begin to reel off their names – Derek, who's been next door for forty years, the Robinsons, the Shelbournes, Marshs ('They've been there years, you know'), Vince, 'who's it Smith', the Packers. 'There's still quite a few,' Sandra muses, although when grandma died nobody collected for her. Now they're putting 'right thieves and trouble-makers' on the street. Muriel was the only trouble-maker before. Everyone knew her and her ways. Sometimes children would call her names to make her mad, just as Sandra and Maggie had once 'shouted quiet like' from their bedroom window at a woman down the road who was 'like Muriel . . . just silly'. But there was no victimisation of the family, no shunning of them, no ridicule. The two sisters grew up feeling safe and accepted in a neigh-bourhood where they were not always having to run for cover.

Such rootedness was not typical of the families in our study. Many others were preyed on by their neighbours, ground down by persistent harassment and forced into a barricaded existence or frequent moves in an effort to escape. The Burgess' experience recounted in chapter 9 makes the contrast. The important point about the sister's story is that it shows how the street community can help to shore up families as surely as it can undo them. Indeed, it was noticeable when locating our subjects how clusters of families were often found in the old mining villages of the South Yorkshire and Derbyshire coalfields.

The grandma factor

Grandma was the linchpin of the family. She 'packed up work to look after Sandra' when she was born. When Maggie arrived some four-and-a-half years later there was talk of her being adopted but 'grandma took one look, she couldn't do it'. Both sisters still remember the ambulance drawing up outside 'when Muriel brought our Tracey home from hospital'. Thirteen years separate Sandra and Tracey so by this time 'grandma were getting on and she wasn't well'. She 'wasn't going to let her bring this last one home, our Tracey. . . . She was definitely not having Tracey.' But when the ambulance drew up she'd 'no choice'. Maggie, who switches between calling her 'grandma' and 'mama', says bluntly, 'mama's always brought us up, you know. . . . Grandma was our mother.'

Having some other adult to turn to is a known factor protecting children in the absence of responsive parents (McIntyre, White and Yoast, 1990; Watt *et al.*, 1995). Grandparents are often the first to step in when affection, support or guidance is missing from the home. The presence or absence of such a positive relationship with grandparents, or some other caring adult, was an important fact differentiating the childhood experience of people in our study. In Maggie and Sandra's case, grandma became a surrogate parent to the extent of usurping Muriel's role as a mother. Grandparents didn't have to take over in order to do their bit. Donald Busby and his mother lived with her parents when he was a child. Donald slept in the front bedroom with 'grandma on that side and granddad on that side and I remaining up in the middle' until he was five or six. Tina Wimpenny used to sleep at her grandma's next door because there 'wasn't enough room at my mam's'. Tracy Talbot's mother spent a lot of time in hospital with thrombosis and whenever she was away the rest of the family, including her father who has learning difficulties, used to move in with the grandparents over the road. Adam Lloyd lived with his mother and grandparents as a boy. He slept in the same room as his mother but it was always his granddad who took him downstairs and rocked him to sleep when he was disturbed. Most families coped better and some only coped at all because there was a grandparent on the scene. Grandparents were undoubtedly a source of resilience in children and when they were not there to call on families had to struggle all the harder to survive.

The parent–child relationship

Maggie and Sandra rail against Muriel for not being the mother they wanted. They refer to her only by her first name: 'We've never called her mam,' Sandra says. 'She never has been, has she, never been a mother?' 'You can't say she's been a mother,' Maggie replies. They always send her a Mother's day card, of course, but Sandra admits she 'won't put "To Mum" in it', only 'To Muriel'.

Muriel has been a constant source of embarrassment and exasperation to her daughters throughout their lives. Maggie frankly admits, 'That's the biggest thing, embarrassed, embarrassed of her.' Always having to explain, always having to warn people, never being sure how she would behave or what she might do. 'She winds you up that much, doesn't she? She winds us all, every one of us, everybody.' 'She does,' agrees Sandra, 'She puts you all on edge.'

Maggie freely confesses that she 'wouldn't be seen out with her at one time'. 'It's only this last few years,' since her grandma died, 'that I've been a bit better.' She recalls how the first time she went shopping with her mother, 'I thought, oh God, please don't let me meet anybody.' Even now she'd 'never take her' to the local market town where she has friends. Sandra chips in, 'We're always threatening her. . . . As we're walking along we can be saying, "I'm telling you, you don't speak to nobody that you shouldn't do", you know.' Maggie suspects that if she bumped into her in the company of a new friend, 'I'd avoid her, I would avoid her.'

Yet the sisters' lives are still intimately bound up with their mother's. They remain in closer touch with her than many daughters who are not so honest about their feelings. It was Muriel who decided to move out of the family home a year after grandma. 'I felt awful,' said Maggie, 'I thought, God, everybody thinks I've kicked her out, but it was Muriel.' She still pops in 'three and four times a week'. Looking back, Maggie says,

I have been bad with her. I mean, I used to say, I hate you, you're not my mother. I used to say it all the time. But then I thought to myself, no, you don't hate her, and you don't really, Sandra, not deep down. I don't really say it now, do I?

Sandra nodded her agreement. 'Muriel's who she is, I should accept that.' Sandra too struggles with her own feelings: 'I feel, I don't feel as though I've got. . . . I mean I feel as though I've got no love for her.' Challenged directly though she's in no doubt that she 'wouldn't want her not to be here. No, I wouldn't want her not here. Oh no, no.' 'It'd be horrible without her,' Maggie added.

Both sisters recognise that they 'aggravate' their mother. 'We've not treated her right,' says Sandra. 'We have treated her wrong,' echoes Maggie. Putting herself in her mother's place, Maggie concedes she would have felt her own behaviour as rejection, 'I would, I would.' For all they slam their mother, they are still protective of her and neither will tolerate people who treat her badly: 'If they wouldn't accept her or take the mickey, then I wouldn't be close to them . . . if they can't accept her then that's their problem, they're no friend.' To which Maggie adds, 'If anybody harmed her, I'd kill them.'

While denying Muriel as their mother the sisters demand she acknowledge them as her daughters. Sandra complains bitterly that the birthday card Muriel sent her was just a plain one, 'not even one with "Daughter" on'. Aside from a friend, Muriel was the only person who rang to wish her happy birthday. Even so, 'I do think I'm last,' says Sandra, admitting 'it hurts, it does'. She feels her mother always 'thought less for me than any of the others': 'I'll just wait till Maggie's birthday and see if she gets a card with "Daughter" on.' Maggie herself shows a similar jealous need for her mother's approval. The fact that Sandra sometimes got more Christmas presents still rankles with her. Even now, 'I might not come off with owt and she might get a present.' She'd recently blown up at her mother for buying her aunts, Muriel's sisters, a present: 'I says I've done with you. I says me and Sandra get bugger all, you know.'

The relationship between Muriel and her two elder daughters reveals many of the same emotions and tensions that are found between most parents and children. There is the same combination of loyalty and rejection, distance and togetherness, give and take, loathing and love, even if they come with a dramatic accent. The plain fact is, though, that it is impossible to conceive of them without each other, and that is both the force and the significance of their story.

Resilience

Maggie and Sandra found different ways of coping with their upbringing. Maggie ran wild. From the time of her grandfather's death, when she was about ten, up to her taking on greater responsibilities in the home as her grandma's health failed, she herself says she 'went off rails': 'I were terrible. I'm ashamed the things I've done. Awful.' Now full of regrets, she offers no excuses for her behaviour. 'I know what I was when I were a kid, and I've always said that if I'd been grandma I'd have had me put away. I would, I would have had me put away. Because I were that bad.' Her sister chips in tersely, 'She was a sod, you know.'

Where Maggie rebelled, Sandra withdrew. Indeed, Maggie's bullying was the main reason why Sandra packed her bags and left the family home to live with her cousin. 'I always used to be frightened of her. She used to belt me, she did. And she'd hit you with anything.' Sandra acknowledges that she 'was always the sort of wimpy one'. She would never have dared do the things her sister did. She remembers once getting a belting from her aunt for smoking on the rec: 'I never had another go.' She describes herself as being, 'all for easy life'. Maggie puts a different gloss on this aspect of her character: 'You let people walk all over you.' Sandra knows that she 'bottles things up'. 'I can't speak my mind like Maggie can. I hold my feelings in. I've got to be really, really wound and wound up before I explode.' Distancing herself from her family was Sandra's way of dealing with the tensions at home. She got back on speaking terms when, pregnant, she had found a new emotional anchorage and a new home with her boyfriend.

Although brought up in the same family, Maggie and Sandra faced a different set of risks and responded in their own individual way. Maggie links her rebelliousness to her unhappiness at not having a dad and her mother being like she is: 'I think my whatsit were with Muriel.' 'That's never bothered me,' Sandra quickly interjects. Maggie was the cause of her trouble: 'As I got to sixteen, as I left school, she was a swine.' Both sisters played an active part in making their own destiny: Sandra by removing herself from the scene of her troubles and Maggie by accepting greater personal responsibility as her grandma's health failed.

Nowadays, when Maggie bumps into people she used to know at school, 'they'll say, God, haven't you changed, quietened down'. She remembers when 'a lot of people wouldn't let their kids play with me'. The Shelbournes included. But David Shelbourne has 'been in nick and all lot and I think to myself, well, I've turned out a hell of a lot better than a lot of them'.

Empty schooldays

Both sisters hated school. The 'school bobby' was a regular visitor at their house. Other children 'used to call' their mother and they found it very hard to put up with the teasing and ridicule. Running away seemed to make sense. The hardest thing was making new friends as they moved through school. Sandra stuck with more or less the same group all the way through from junior school because 'they all knew her, so they was all right with her'. Maggie too found it difficult having 'to start over again' every time she made new friends. Once they got to secondary school 'there was only a few people that knew about Muriel'. It was easier to keep it that way by not bringing people home, except for those 'who knew her and what she was'. While they used to go round other's houses, they 'never had any people stopping here'. Having to explain was too embarrassing. Maggie recalls going on a school exchange visit to Bournemouth. When the time came for them to host the return, 'I remember they had to go to a friend's house, Jill's, and didn't have them here. Can't have one here cos of Muriel.' Perhaps a legacy of the necessary restraint they learned to adopt with other children is that neither Maggie or Sandra have many friends their own age. Sandra prefers the company of older people while Maggie says, 'I've clung to my animals.'

Lack of demonstrable affect

Maggie remembers the first real hug her mother gave her. It was when grandma died. She was twenty-three. But then the family were never brought up to show their feelings. 'I mean we must have had love, but we was never, I don't know, we wasn't like hugged all the time.' Neither sister can recall ever seeing their grandparents show any affection to each other or to any of their own daughters, including Muriel. 'We're not like that, are we?', says Sandra. 'No,' answers Maggie, 'It's somewhere from a long time ago that's gone wrong, and it's passed on to all of us.' Muriel's older sister, their aunt, is just the same: 'she can't go and hug her own daughters'. Maggie recalls an episode when their cousin Ethel nearly lost her husband: 'She was crying. There was me, her two sisters, her dad and mam, and not one went to comfort her.' Maggie feels she has 'learnt to be that bit more loving where Sandra won't, will you?' 'No,' comes the blunt reply. 'I don't think it's right to be like we are,' Maggie adds ruefully.

Low self-esteem

'I've always been one to pull myself down,' confesses Sandra, 'I think I can't do it before I've even had a go.' Maggie admitted to having the same chronic self-doubts: 'I've got no confidence in myself. I always think people are better than me.' They attribute some of these feelings to 'Muriel being as she is'. Their embarrassment about their mother has left them vulnerable in the world, always thinking that other people have got something over them. But Muriel is by no means the only factor in the equation. Under-achievement at school also plays a part. 'I always say I'm thick,' says Sandra. The only activities they enjoyed or felt to be any good at were sport and community service. Their basic literacy skills suffered as a result of persistent absenteeism which their grandma colluded in and even encouraged. The fear of being shown up in class – of being unable to answer the teacher – has carried through into their adult lives. Poverty too helped to stiffen their sense of inferiority. They never had a family holiday. Sandra recalls her second-hand clothes. Maggie had her hand-me-downs. 'We never had like people at school.' Their clothes were always just going out of fashion. 'I hated that,' says Maggie, 'Like my mates'd go out. Sharon, you can guarantee she'd have proper fashion, and I'd be like one step behind her. That's . . . always better than me . . . that's why I probably think people are always better than me.' The only time she remembers being modish was 'when it were punk rock and you just wore everything scruffy'.

The social production of (in)competence

Muriel's life has been shaped by the people around her as surely as it has by her learning difficulties. Lacking skills perhaps, she has also been de-skilled by her family and by the support services. Maggie recognises the truth of the matter: Muriel, she says, has been 'mollycoddled'. Grandma has 'always done for her' and 'all family's not helped' by falling into line. Sandra backs her up: 'Grandma, she did everything. She never really let her do anything.' Since Muriel moved out of the family home into Social Services accommodation, Maggie sees it all happening over again: 'They've ruined her as well.'

Grandma took over Muriel's parental role: 'Grandma was our mother.' She put a stop to Muriel's relationship with the sisters' father and brought them up 'never to have nothing to do with him'. (Although whatever was between their parents has stood the test of time. There are four-and-a-half years between Maggie and Sandra, and Muriel is now in touch with their father again some thirty and more years on.) Grandma controlled all Muriel's money: 'she's never, ever had money, only a bit of spending money'. When Muriel put in for a house of her own some years back, and was offered a tenancy in Triangle Crescent, it was grandma who said she didn't want her to go and persuaded her to turn it down. Maggie now suspects that her one-time violent and aggressive behaviour was a side effect of the drugs she was on. And when grandma began to fail and needed looking after, the family accepted the offer of a place in an Adult Training Centre for Muriel even though they knew she 'shouldn't be with them sort of people' and 'doesn't belong there at all'.

Alongside the evidence of chances in life lost or denied are to be found the signs of competencies never fully brought out or realised. Muriel 'started off at a normal school' but was later sent away to a residential place in Buxton ('I can remember mama saying there was grown-up people walking round with dolls.'). Like many people with learning difficulties, she came to parenthood without the experience of an ordinary family life. Somewhere along the way she learned to read, write, count and handle money. She is also streetwise: as Maggie says, she 'can get anywhere' and 'find anybody'. When Tracey ran off with her boyfriend and went missing for months, leaving her sisters chasing round in circles with worry, it was Muriel who had the nous to leave a message for her at the dole office. Indeed she has always shown a maternal interest in the welfare of her children. It was Muriel who used to take and meet them from school until they were old enough to find their own way, and who took them to the doctor's, and the dentist's: 'She always took us to things like that more than grandma', says Sandra. Maggie told of how she'd had 'bent fingers' as a child and her mother had arranged to have them corrected in hospital: 'It wasn't right for Muriel, I wasn't perfect. She made me go and have them done.' Although the hospital was in another town, Muriel had taken her in on the bus and was the only person to visit her. The sisters' cousin Angie has noticed how Muriel is 'always there' whenever anyone from the family is in hospital: 'I had my tonsils out, I was only in for two days. Muriel still found her way down, and found the ward. Nobody'd told her.' Indeed, Muriel shows herself to be a family person in all sorts of ways. She 'never misses a birthday, never'. She's always giving little presents, often without a word of thanks in return. As Maggie observes, 'heart's there, you know'. Tellingly, when Maggie blew up in a fit of jealousy because she felt left out, Muriel brought her a poinsettia the next day. She gets on well with her grandson, William, who 'has always accepted her as yet' – 'You want to see them playing football together down garden!' – and she's bought her baby granddaughter, Katherine, 'all sorts of little bits of things'. When Maggie was suffering a lot of back trouble and couldn't go to work, she asked Muriel to stay over for a week and look after her (having always turned to grandma when she was ill as a child): 'She was as good as gold, she couldn't do enough. And I'd do it again, if I wasn't very well. I'd ask her and she'd love it.'

Both sisters are intuitively aware of spent possibilities in Muriel's life. She 'used to get on at work . . . she were pretty good'. She particularly liked her job as an office cleaner. Maggie remembers 'playing about with phone pressing numbers' when Muriel took them with her. Both think she might have managed in her own house at this time given some help with budgeting. They see the parallels with their younger sister. Tracey's also 'backward . . . summat like a thirteen-year-old and she's twenty' and inclined to throw 'a bit of a tantrum': 'She's a lot like Muriel,' says Sandra. When Tracey left special school they found her a job with them 'and she was as right as rain, no problems' until she got laid off. Then 'it started . . . because she'd got nowt to do . . . different friends and stopping out all night' until finally she upped and left to set up home with her boyfriend. Since Katherine was born they can see the difference in her: 'she's grown up more with baby'. Muriel was never allowed to demonstrate her competence in the same way. 'She'd be a different person to be honest', broods Maggie.

The cultural ambivalence of parenthood

Parenthood challenges the myth of the eternal child that pervades social attitudes towards people with learning difficulties. Becoming a parent marks the final transition to a fully adult status in society. Having learning difficulties usually means being assigned a Peter Pan role in life and an identity to match. The conjunction of the two generates the sort of moral uncertainty and social ambiguity that always arises when the boundaries between deeply ingrained cultural categories are compromised or crossed. The parent with learning difficulties presents as a kind of living contradiction: the adult child, the knowing innocent, the chaste lover, the dependent carer, the blind watchman. Uncertainty about how to categorise people tends to lead to inconsistencies in the way others behave towards them. Such inconsistencies are evident in the relationship the two sisters have with their mother, and in the frustrations experienced by Muriel herself.

As a mother and grandmother, Muriel is still treated like a child by her own daughters who are constantly reprimanding and chastising her about her behaviour, about what she wears, about how she does her hair:

> She come down on Friday. Her hair looked a mess. She'd got socks on with trainers, you keep telling her off for that. She just doesn't try, does she? Then she'll come down with black tights on and white trainers. You can't tell her.

Denied her maternal role, she is nevertheless expected to behave like a mother. Maggie comments disapprovingly on her 'liking for the lads' ('She was a bugger') but admits she was probably no different to any other unmarried, sexually active woman: 'But then again, you don't, I mean Muriel's a parent, isn't she?' Never having had any money of her own ('She only had pocket money'), Muriel is still expected to be bountiful: 'I mean you never get nothing really decent off her, like any other parent.' Cast in the dependent role of service user and receiver of care in her adult foster placement ('Bob, he does everything') and the training centre ('She's always complaining about it'), Muriel is also required to play the part of carer within her own family if the need arises, as when Maggie hurt her back.

Sometimes the contradictory demands and expectations foisted on Muriel drive her to breaking-point. Forced to allow Sandra to do her hair, 'she just started in one of her moods'. One or two incidents recounted by the sisters suggest that Muriel was sensitive about having her maternal role taken away. Maggie recalls once how she had started putting Tracey in an old Silver Cross pram from out of the garden shed: 'Grandma says you mustn't put that baby in it, it's damp. And she flung out at grandma, blacked her eye.' On another occasion, again when Tracey was a baby, Muriel had flown at her sister Ann's then boyfriend, later her husband, for saying coochie-coo to the baby: 'She said, "She's not effing well yours." She went crazy, crazy.'

The culturally ambivalent position of parents such as Muriel makes it hard for both them and others to negotiate a balance between what Harrington and Whiting (1972) have described as the attributed aspects of their identity (those assigned by the wider society), its subjective components (how individuals think others see them), and its optative features (how people would like others to see them). A 'healthy identity' has these three factors in balance (Angrosino, 1998). The sisters' story illustrates the tensions that can arise in relationships when they are out of sync.

Misdirected support

The Lewis family received little in the way of practical support from the statutory services while Maggie and Sandra were growing up. 'There weren't no social workers when we was little . . .', Sandra says, with Maggie quickly adding, ' . . . and there ought to have been with me'. Apart from anything else, grandma 'wouldn't have anybody in house'. Maggie remembers how 'grandma kicked them out once. They come to door and I says, "I'm sorry I can't let you in", and we got rid of them. Just tried to cope on us own.'

It was only as grandma grew older, and Tracey, their younger sister, became more 'unruly', that the family began to feel the need for help. 'It all started from Mrs Kessingland', Maggie recalls. 'She used to bring clothes. I think Mrs Kessingland got grandma help.' Tracey was fostered twice, and periodically 'they'd send Muriel to Bank House for a fortnight'. Mostly though, it 'were just lecturing'. 'I don't think there was as much help as we wanted', Maggie reflects. 'With grandma being old, and Muriel being as she is as well, I think they could have done a bit more.'

All the support the family received was targeted on grandma as the 'carer' rather than Muriel as the mother of three young children. The services only stepped in, and the door only opened to them, when old age and infirmity whittled away grandma's ability to cope. No effort was made to support Muriel in her parenting at any time. Indeed, she was defined as part of the problem. Up to the point when she finally chose to leave the family home, after grandma had died, the only services Muriel ever received were provided against her wishes for the benefit of others. She was sent to the Adult Training Centre, at the suggestion of social services, to get her out of the way during the day although, as Sandra admits, 'She's always complaining about it.' Likewise, every now and then she was packed off into respite accommodation 'to give mama a break', although she 'used to play up terrible' before she went, shouting 'I'm not going, I'm not going.'

Help for the family usually came at Muriel's expense. Her needs as a parent were never acknowledged or addressed. The services responded to grandma as a carer and Muriel as a client. When the strains began to mount in the home, their answer was to remove Muriel rather than to see how the family might be supported as a unit. As Maggie says about her going to the training centre, 'We didn't say we want her putting there.' But then, for 'the welfare' as for the family, Muriel was always her mother's daughter rather than her daughters' mother.

Distributed competence

Let's be clear about the achievements of the Lewis family. Three generations have grown up or grown old in the same house. The years have brought them their share of troubles: a grandfather crippled and slowly suffocating from the coal dust in his lungs; a daughter and granddaughter (as well as a mother and sister) with learning difficulties; for grandma, an adult life of uninterrupted child-rearing ending only when age and arthritis rendered her in need of support herself; a delinquent teenager out of control; for Maggie, responsibilities at a young age for the care of her beloved, ageing grandmother; domestic overcrowding; and always, always the spoiling effects of poverty. Yet they have come through, as a family, together, with almost no outside support, apart from the kindness of neighbours, and only their own resourcefulness, love and humour on which to draw, so that Sandra can still say, 'I can never remember being unhappy.'

Their story illustrates an exemplary point: competence is rarely if ever a solo performance. Competence as a property is a feature of social relationships rather than people as individuals. It is, as Bruner (1990, 1991) might put it, both *situated* in an individual's social network and *distributed* across that network. From this position it is not surprising to find that 'the presence of a tightly-knit social network was positively associated with parents' sense of competence in parenting' (Webster-Stratton, 1990). Among other things, such networks provide practical assistance to parents, options for the temporary or permanent redistribution of children, and a context for sharing, validating and enforcing standards of child-care (Korbin, 1987).

In Muriel's case, her close family network helped to compensate for her own limitations as a mother in order to secure the welfare of her children through their passage into adulthood. Only Tracey spent any time outside the care of the family, when she was fostered a couple of times to give grandma a short break. The other side of this achievement is that Muriel's embeddedness in her family came at the cost of her own independence. The price of meeting the needs of her children was the loss of her role as a mother. Taking a situated approach to competence, we might say there was an imbalance in the distribution of responsibilities within the family that limited Muriel's capacity to fulfil her part as a mother as well as she might have done given the opportunity to show what she could do.

The themes untangled above are not special to Maggie and Sandra's story. They have been highlighted precisely because they recur as topics throughout the accounts of the people in our study. Of course, they receive a slightly different spin in other tales. But though the cloth may vary the cut remains the same. Following Erikson (1973) we have tried to show how the particular features of the sisters' narrative can be subsumed under more general headings. For all its uniqueness, Sandra and Maggie's experience is structured by the same forces that help to shape the lives of other people with similar parents. These forces are revealed not as facts to be counted or rendered by numbers but as incidents and episodes sharing a similar dramatic purpose in people's narratives. By analysing Maggie and Sandra's story carefully, we have tried to show these forces at work in order to establish its emblematic stature.

NARRATIVE AS METHOD

Narrative is both a source of data about 'lives in the world' and a means of producing stories about those lives. Acknowledging this distinction between events-as-lived and events-as-told raises the question, posed by Plummer (1990), of 'what is the link between the life itself and its story?' This question directs attention to the process by which accounts of lives are produced and turned into text. In this section we explore two problematic aspects of this process: what Lincoln and Denzin (1994) have called the issue of *representation* and the issue of *legitimation*. The issue of representation is about the authenticity of the experience reported in the text. The issue of legitimation is about the authority of the text and our claims for its verisimilitude. Both issues go to the heart of the narrative method and have a direct bearing on what we make of Maggie and Sandra's story.

Whose story is it anyway?

Research narratives are almost always the product of more than one author: usually a subject (as narrator) and a researcher (as rapporteur). They are properly seen as 'the creation of two minds working together' (Whittemore, Langness and Koegel, 1986). It is rarely possible to determine whether the questions shaped the story or the story shaped the questions.

Clandinin and Connelly (1994) point out that in translating the raw material generated by field research into a publishable story the researcher puts himself or herself into the text. Deciding how to 'be there in the text' (Geertz, 1988) presents one of the most difficult decisions facing the narrative researcher. It involves striking a balance between the researcher's and the subject's frame of reference. At one extreme, the researcher may adopt the role of an amanuensis (whose contribution adds nothing to the meaning of the text); at the other, a biographer (who writes about the lives of others in the third person). The researcher adds his or her own signature to the story whatever balance is finally struck along this continuum. At this point, it becomes the researcher's as well as the subject's story.

Maggie and Sandra's story is recounted entirely in the first person, but its origins are not just in their own imagination and experience. It also comes out of the research relationship that led to its telling. People provide different versions of who they are at different points in their lives and assemble their past in different ways for different audiences (Maines, 1993). Storied lives are under constant revision. There is no fixed biographical truth awaiting discovery by the conscientious researcher, only a 'shifting web of meanings' (Plummer, 1990). Maggie and Sandra might have had something different to say if they had been seen separately, or if their younger cousin had not sat in on a couple of the sessions, or if Sandra's son had not come into the room when she was talking about his relationship with his grandma, or if they had been interviewed by someone else (say a man instead of a woman). The account presented in the previous chapter is an account of their story as told under the specific conditions of its narration, and as such it owes something to the sisters' relationship with the researcher as surely as it does to their recollections of a shared past.

Allowing that people may honestly present different versions of their own past means that narrative inconsistency cannot be taken as evidence of unreliability or deception. However, it does raise the problem for the researcher of deciding which facets of self are being emphasised or underplayed. The fact that Maggie and Sandra were interviewed together, and much of their story developed as a dialogue, limited their scope for shamming or for electing how to present themselves. One was always ready to pull the other up if she deviated from their jointly remembered past. Thus when Sandra said of Maggie, 'She was a sod, you know', Maggie was obliged to acknowledge that aspect of her character when she was growing up. In a similar vein, narrative researchers may pick up, articulate, and develop aspects of people's stories to create identities that serve their purposes but do not match their subjects' sense of who they are. This is an ever-present danger of the common method of 'exampling' by which carefully selected extracts from life stories are used to support a narrative of the researcher's own making. By contrast, the practice of what has been called 'thick description' – writing at length and in detail about a specific case – which we employed in the previous chapter, where the subjects' voices remain dominant throughout, makes it almost impossible to impose a point of view that rubs against the grain of the story.

The issue of whose voice we are hearing in Maggie and Sandra's story arises in another guise too. Our interest is in our subjects' experience of growing up. Unable to track anyone step-by-step as they negotiated the transition into adulthood, we followed Maggie and Sandra retrospectively through autobiographical reflection. All such narratives are told in the present even when their focus is the past. Maggie and Sandra's story is related by them as adults, but features them as children. Does this make it the adults' or the children's story? Is the child speaking *through* the adult or is the adult speaking *for* the child? Are Maggie and Sandra interpreting their childhood experience from a position in the adult world or recounting what they felt as children? Whyte (1996) observes that informants' memories of earlier events 'are inevitably clouded by what has been happening to them in the intervening years'. For this reason, Clandinin and Connelly (1994) conclude that memory unaided by contemporary sources usually expresses a 'current voice'. We are not so sure. When Maggie recalls not wanting her mother to meet her out of school, she is clearly evoking her embarrassment at the time, not projecting later feelings onto an earlier self. What is perhaps significant is that this embarrassment has remained with her into adult life. In other words, it is not the provenance of the childhood memories that is at stake but their meaning for the adult reporting them.

Maggie and Sandra's story is as much about their mother as themselves, although Muriel herself plays only a walk-on part in its narration. It is not Muriel's story but it is about Muriel. She would undoubtedly present herself in a different light, and give a different account of the same happenings. The portrait is that of a mother as seen by her daughters. If the result is unfair to Muriel as a person it does not render the sisters' narrative any the less true to their own experience.

Some people have called for an 'ethics of representation' that would require narrative researchers to make clear who is speaking in their texts (Abrams, 1991). The arguments rehearsed above show that such an ideal may be hard to achieve. Perhaps a more workable test is whether the narrator is prepared to acknowledge ownership of the story. The sisters were sent a draft for comment. The fact that Maggie chose to dedicate the chapter to her grandma gives us confidence that she recognised herself in the text.

Writing stories

The spoken word does not easily transfer onto the printed page. Speech and prose do not share the same grammar. We mostly do not talk in sentences. We use pitch and movement and stress to divide up chunks of meaning. Turning transcripts into publishable scripts calls for editorial intervention. Even a master of the medium of talk like Alaistair Cooke (1980) confesses to 'making the most of the privilege of print to straighten out the syntax' of his broadcasts in the published collections of his *Letters from America*. The issue for the narrative researcher is how far an editor can mess with the words of informants before the quest for intelligibility threatens the integrity of the text (Booth, 1995).

Every word in the sisters' narrative was spoken by them, excepting only some necessary changes in proper names in order to preserve confidentiality, some judicious insertion of 'marker' phrases to identify who is speaking for the reader, and some use of 'Parkerisms' (see below). Nevertheless, their published story bears only a passing resemblance to the full transcripts of the interviews. Several techniques were used to create the continuous dialogue that forms their narrative.

Compression

Compression involves cutting and pasting quotations from different parts of an interview, or from interviews with the same subject(s) conducted at different times, into a single monologue.

People rarely wrap up a topic in one go or tell a story from beginning to end during depth interviews. They may lose their flow, get side-tracked, raise something in passing that the interviewer is able to pick up only later, recall additional material at a later point, or choose to disclose more as trust develops. A new question may prompt different memories, the interview may be interrupted (by a crying baby, a knock at the door, the telephone), people repeat things. For these and other reasons, stories do not usually emerge fully formed, but in snatches. The act of narration rarely follows a straight course. Compression is a means of giving coherence to stories in the making.

Elision

In everyday discourse, people frequently make false starts and repeated attempts at expressing what they want to say. Elision refers to the running together of passages that were separated by such superfluous material in the transcript in order to better convey their sense. Take, for example, the following verbatim sentence spoken by Maggie: 'To think that I'd had me, my sister had got to be fostered out.' This line would be more clearly phrased, without causing the reader to stumble, and without twisting Maggie's words as: 'To think that my sister had got to be fostered out.' Elisions ease the flow of the text without any change of meaning or any change of voice.

Splicing

Splicing involves merging adjacent passages spoken by the same person that were separated by extraneous material in the transcript. The main reason for splicing is to maintain the coherence of the storyline and the dramatic flux of the narrative.

Consider, for example, the following extract from one of the interviews in which Maggie is talking about how she always has to tell other people that her mother's condition was caused *in utero* when grandma contracted double pneumonia:

Maggie: . . . (it) caused Muriel to be backward. The doctor told grandma don't buy all these things because there may not be any baby. That's what, and I've always had to go right into that.

Int: Was she on some medication that caused it then? I mean, if she had double pneumonia, was she made to take something?

Maggie: I don't know if she was or not. She had double pneumonia and they always say that's what she made Muriel like she is.

Sandra: Well, it's harder in them days wasn't it.

Maggie: That's what I've always had to explain to people. I've had to go right through it. So I wouldn't feel so bad. I wouldn't like say well, Muriel's backward, I'd have to go all the way through it to blame double pneumonia just for it.

This exchange was edited by splicing and attributed to Maggie in the final text, as it appears in the previous chapter, as follows:

Maggie: . . . caused Muriel to be backward. The doctor told grandma don't buy all these things because there may not be any baby.

> That's what I've always had to explain to people. I've had to
> go right through it, so I wouldn't feel so bad. I wouldn't, like,
> say, well, Muriel's backward. I'd have to go all the way
> through it to blame double pneumonia for it.

The final passage also shows some minor changes in punctuation when
compared with the transcript. Speech does not contain commas or full
stops. The punctuation in the transcript has been inserted by the audio-
typist when transcribing the tapes. The researcher as editor should not
be misled into thinking that the typed copy somehow represents the raw
narrative. In preparing the text, the transcript will require careful revision to catch the rhythm, inflection, stress, and sense of the original
voice.

Omission

The complete transcripts of the three interviews with Maggie and
Sandra run to some 28,000 words. The final text which appears in
chapter 6 is just short of 11,000 words in length. Clearly, even allowing
for elision and splicing, a lot of words have been lost on the way. The
excised material mostly falls into one of the following categories of
data: *repetition* (a normal feature of extended interviews spread over a
matter of weeks); *irrelevancies* (meaning material that does not add to an
understanding of the sisters' past or present such as, for example,
passing conversation about Sandra's son's migraines); *interrogative material*
(where the sisters sought to clarify with each other the precise nature of
the facts or the sequence of events as a prelude to articulating their
answer to a question); *expendable trivia* (like chit-chat about the problems
Sandra's husband is having with their car or Maggie's ambition to own
some miniature horses); *self-registering material* (in the form of, for
example, questions put by the sisters to the interviewer, or other material emanating from the researcher or referring to the research); and
other kinds of *conversational packaging*.

Erasing the questions

The erasure of the interviewer's questions constitutes an important,
specific case of omission. The researcher has been taken out of the text
(other than as the hidden hand editing the material). The aim is not
artifice – to pretend that the sisters' dialogue is something it is not. The
purpose is to focus attention on Maggie and Sandra as people rather

than on the interview as a process. In this respect, we have followed the example of Tony Parker as an acknowledged master of tape-recorded speech. Parker liked to think of himself as no more than 'a blackboard for people to write on' (Thompson, 1994). Self-effacement was a key part of his technique for breathing life into his characters. Another typical Parkerism we have adopted is occasionally to embody the question in the subject's response (Garfield, 1995) as a way of putting over information while maintaining the narrative flow or signalling a change of topic.

Time

We have already referred to the distinction between events-as-lived and events-as-told. Implicit in this distinction is a recognition that accounts of lives may not have the same temporal structure as lived experience. Lives are lived out in chronological time where the past always precedes the present, the order of things is fixed, and the future never comes. Accounts of lives take place in story-time in which the narrator is free to roam backwards and forwards through history and to rearrange the relationship between past, present and future.

A further distinction may also be drawn between story-time and discourse-time, where the former refers to the ordering of material in the narrative and the latter refers to the ordering of material in the text. The sequencing and pacing of stories as recounted reflect the conditions of their narration. A sudden interruption – a knock at the door, someone entering the room, a baby crying – may force a break in the interview and bring about a change of topic. Later questions may yield further information about a subject discussed earlier. The interviewer may decide to back off on a stressful topic for a while and pick it up again later. Such factors – which influence how a story comes to be disclosed – are not necessarily the ones that should determine how it is reported. They also remind us that there is nothing sacrosanct about the arrangement of material in the transcript. It is the product of the interviewer (who asked the questions) as much as the respondent (who provided the answers).

Three specific techniques were used to create the time-frame of Maggie and Sandra's story. Material was transposed by moving it backwards or forwards relative to where it appeared in the transcript. The tense of some verbs was changed where not to have done might have confused the reader. Breaks were inserted in the text which do not correspond to breaks in the interviews, and the interviews themselves were treated as one continuous dialogue.

Emplotment

Keeping in mind the whole picture while finding a way through the flood of detail that washes through the transcripts is one of the most difficult tasks facing the narrative researcher. Finding a slant or perspective for giving coherence to the chaotic press of raw material is a crucial step in this process. Bowen (1968) has described it as 'plotting the biography'. By setting limits on what the reader sees of the life portrayed, emplotment performs much the same function in narrative as theory does in empirical research (Walker, 1981).

Our interest in the sisters centred on their relationship with their mother. We have no doubt that this relationship was a defining feature of their lives and had a profound influence on their sense of self. At the same time, we cannot be sure that Muriel would be given the same prominence in the stories they might tell to other listeners. Stories use emplotment to convey a point. In Maggie and Sandra's case, their story is organised around a plot of our choosing.

Faraday and Plummer (1979) warn us never to forget that in narrative research there is always much more to the story than we are getting. At the same time, the process of turning interviews into text inevitably entails leaving stuff out. Caught between these twin diktats of the method, narrative researchers always risk betraying their subjects in the act of representing them. In putting together the sisters' story we have tried to live up to Victoria Glendinning's description of a biographer as a novelist under oath. Our approach has been governed by two precepts: honesty (in our dealings with Maggie and Sandra, in our use of material and to our readers) and readability. One way of ensuring a degree of accountability for the final text is for us to reveal the part we have played in its production. In this section, we have tried to fulfil this obligation.

Chapter 8

The myth of the upside down family

In this chapter we examine the idea of role reversal as a feature of relationships between disabled parents and their children. Children, so the reasoning goes, drawn into making good their disabled parents' limitations, frequently end up by stepping into their shoes. Using the personal narratives of the now-adult children in our study, we shall argue that this picture amounts to a caricature that seriously misrepresents the impact of disability on family life.

The notion of role reversal has been most fully developed recently in the context of discussion about the 'lost childhood' of young carers. The term 'young carer' denotes a new welfare category. It refers to the situation of children and young people who are obliged to assume prime responsibility for the care of an ill or disabled parent, to the point of becoming 'the guardian of their own parent's welfare' (Aldridge and Becker, 1993). These caring responsibilities go well beyond the kind of duties that children might normally be expected to perform within the family. Note how a social worker who now works with a young carers' group defines the difference: 'helping out in a family is fine but being a young carer is far more than helping out. You are taking on the role of an adult, performing caring tasks which a child shouldn't be expected to do (BBC, 1994)'. This position closely matches that of the Social Services Inspectorate (1995) which has defined a young carer as 'a child or young person who is carrying out significant caring tasks and assuming a level of responsibility for another person, which would usually be taken by an adult.'

These tasks and responsibilities are onerous and extensive enough to turn the family upside down – the young carer 'swopping places' with the parent and effectively becoming 'the adult of the house'. Segal and Simkins (1993) report that many of the children they met who had ill or disabled parents 'believed at times that they looked after their parents, rather than the other way round.'

The young carers debate portrays disabled parents in an almost entirely negative light (Turner, 1995). They are shown as ill-equipped to fulfil their parenting role, and their children are held to suffer as a consequence in two main ways. The first is by having to sacrifice their own childhood in caring for their parents: 'I hated having to be so restricted because I couldn't think of myself. I had to think of my father all the time (a young carer in Turner, 1995)'. Children themselves talk openly about 'having to grow up fast', 'caring emotionally and physically' from an early age, having 'to run a household', 'taking on the role of the housewife', being unable to go out to play, 'missing out on friends', losing 'the years of innocence' and having no 'nice childhood memories' (BBC, 1994).

The burden of caring is also presented as exacting a toll in later life through its effects on child development. The same voices from the BBC radio documentary cited above talk of how: 'You miss out on your education because your schooling is disrupted'; 'You're stigmatised, you're picked on, you're bullied'; 'I couldn't go out and socialise with my peers and because of that (they) looked on me as someone slightly strange, so it set me apart'; 'I didn't get out to meet anybody'; 'It's very lonely. You spend most of your time on your own'; 'It was hard for me to socialise because I've never had to'; it leaves you 'not being able to relate to other people'; 'You grow up without the emotional or psychological tools to deal with things'. Aldridge and Becker (1993) argue that there are clear 'developmental and emotional implications in the long term effects of caring on children' and that a child who is prevented from engaging fully in play, education and social interaction is going to suffer adverse effects in later life.

The validity of the category of young carer and the notion of role reversal have not gone unchallenged. Both have attracted a string of criticisms from disability rights activists and others who question the evidence used to back them up and its interpretation. For a start, deciding precisely who qualifies as a young carer is far from straightforward. This problem accounts for the huge variations found in estimates of their numbers, which range from 40,000 to 200,000 (Tithridge, 1995). Clearly people hold different ideas about how to interpret the kind of definition put forward by the Social Services Inspectorate. This itself is not surprising as there are no norms for children's involvement in running a household or helping out in the family (Webster, 1991). Almost nothing is known about what they do around the house.

Consequently, there is no baseline for fixing the normal expectations against which an undue load might be assessed. Moreover, these expectations change over time with changes in prevailing ideas about the nature of childhood (Ariès, 1979) and vary by culture, class, race, age and gender (Hendrick, 1990; James and Prout, 1990; Jenks, 1982). In practice the task of deciding just when 'helping out' in the family exceeds what should reasonably be expected of a child is a question of judgement rather than a matter of fact. There is no common scale for fixing such a point and no fixed boundary dividing children's rights from adult responsibilities.

These problems are made more difficult because 'young carers' often do not describe themselves in such terms. Consequently, researchers 'have imposed their own definitions and perceptions' on their subjects (Keith and Morris, 1996). This has led to a one-sided emphasis on the downside of life as a young carer and a failure to acknowledge there may be positive aspects to the experience, as this young person recognises: 'In a way I've gained from it. Because I grew up so quickly, now I've got a pretty mature outlook on life. . . . I know what can be achieved and what can't be achieved. So in a way it's helped me. . . .' (BBC, 1994). The attention given to the problems of young carers has also served to represent their experience in purely personal terms. They care because their parent(s) can't. This equation forges a direct link between the burden on the child and the disabilities of the parent. As Aldridge and Becker (1993) explain, 'the nature and extent of the care receiver's illness or disability was a determining factor on the level of caring responsibilities undertaken by the young carers.' This simple correlation begins to break down as soon as one looks beyond the parent's disability, when other factors are often seen to come into play. Take the following case vignette, for example:

> Tina has kidney failure and her husband contributes very little to the family's care needs. They have two daughters, Jane, aged 17, and Alice, aged 9. Jane, despite being in full-time education, does most of the caring tasks for both her mother and sister as well as the housework.
>
> (Bond, 1995)

In this instance, it is the division of labour within the household rather than the mother's disability that makes for Jane's predicament. Jane's father looks to her to take on the domestic and caring aspects of the maternal role in order to preserve his own position in the family. The decision of the (usually male) non-disabled parent to delegate responsibilities in this way often plays a crucial part in determining the caring responsibilities of children (Olsen, 1996). In another scenario, children may be obliged to assume a greater burden in two-parent households where low pay and long hours or other demands of the job mean that the non-disabled partner is out at work for much of the day or frequently away from home. Young people are also known to shoulder more than their share either because their parents are reluctant to seek support in case it leads to the break-up of the family or because they themselves daren't say anything for fear of what outside intervention might bring (Rickford, 1995). Children too are pushed into over-involvement in caring roles because their parents are inadequately supported. Indeed, one of the criticisms of the young carers debate is that the issue has been framed in terms of relieving the burden on children rather than promoting the independence of disabled parents (Parker and Olsen, 1995b). Concentrating attention on the needs of young carers runs the risk of ignoring those environmental, social and economic factors that discriminate against disabled parents and make it more difficult for them to fulfil their parenting role. As Parker and Olsen say, 'If the aim is to give children back their childhood, this may be better achieved by giving parents back their parenthood (Parker and Olsen, 1995a)'.

Role reversal is presented as a characteristic feature of young caring but what it means in practice raises as many questions as the term 'young carer' itself. In truth, there is very little empirical grounding for the idea beyond the observation that in some families and in some circumstances some children and young people assume tasks that would normally be undertaken by a parent. In the literature on young carers, however, the notion of role reversal – or reverse dependency as it has also been called – goes beyond such simple facts to describe a situation where the child 'becomes the parent of the parent' (Aldridge and Becker, 1993), who in turn becomes a dependent of the child. It is at this point that the bobbin starts to unwind.

There is no evidence that young caring leads to any leaching of identity between parent and child. While the customary balance of reciprocity in parent-child relationships may be up-ended by illness or impairment there is nothing to suggest that a corresponding re-negotiation of status takes place. As Fisher (1986) points out, tasks are more easily redistributed than power. She reports that while daughter-respondents used the term role reversal to describe the changing nature of their relationships with their ageing and increasingly frail mothers, none of the mother-respondents did so. A notable feature of much research on young carers is the absence of the parents' viewpoint (for an exception, see Aldridge and Becker, 1994).

Part of the problem with the notion of role reversal stems from the muddled conception of parenthood it embodies. Parenthood is both an identity and a task. As an identity it involves both an officially conferred status and a specific conception of self. As a task it involves a variable set of skills and activities linked to the individual's changing position in the life cycle. The literature on young carers fails properly to distinguish these two aspects of the parenting role. Disability may limit people's capacities to perform some aspects of the parenting task – especially when additional barriers are put in their way through lack of support and public prejudice – but it does not unavoidably spoil their identity as parents. The reality, of course, is that people can and do remain parents without necessarily performing the parental task and, equally, act as parents without becoming parents – that, after all, is what fostering is about. Aldridge and Becker (1993) implicitly acknowledge this distinction in their discussion of the relationship between the disabled parents and young carers when they concede that: 'Pragmatically the roles might have been reversed, but emotionally their parents' status as guardians remained intact.' In this light, talk of children 'parenting their parent' overstates the case and role reversal is seen to be a misnomer. What is really at issue is the redistribution of tasks within the family rather than a wholesale recasting of identities.

An assumption underlying a good deal of the discussion about role reversal in the young carers literature is that disability entails dependency. Requiring help with domestic chores or personal care is equated with handing over responsibility to someone else: needing personal assistance is taken to mean needing to be looked after. Hence the idea that children who take on parenting tasks (such as looking after younger brothers and sisters) also assume parental responsibilities and that children who provide care for their parents thereby acquire responsibility for them. Keith and Morris (1996) point out how 'all disabled parents experience the assumption of strangers that our children "look after" us.' The disability movement has fought hard to challenge this way of thinking by unpicking the cultural association between independence and doing things for oneself. The point, says Brisenden (1989), 'is that independent people have control over their lives, not that they perform every task themselves.' As Morris argues (1993) independence and responsibility are not forfeited when a disabled person retains control over what help is provided, when and how. Interestingly, Aldridge and Becker (1993) report that none of the young or adult carers in their study 'talked about the care receiver in terms of dependency'. Similarly, Segal and Simpkins (1993) found that ' "My dad can't" or "My mum can't" are phrases seldom used by these children'. The fact that disabled parents and their children are able to negotiate the divide between disability and dependency in their everyday lives and routines again suggests that the so-called process of role reversal – or reverse dependency – presents a misreading of family relationships in such households.

Role reversal has mostly been discussed in relation to parents with a physical impairment and their children. There has been much less written about role reversal in families headed by a parent or parents with learning difficulties, partly because there is a smaller body of research in this field and partly too because the bulk of the work done so far has concentrated on parents with very young children (Tymchuk, 1990b). Nevertheless, despite the lack of any firm empirical evidence, there is an assumption running through much of the literature that older children in such families tend either to take over once they out-smart their parents or to run wild. Accardo and Whitman (1990), for example, warn that 'a normal child of a retarded parent may be stressed to assume a "parental child" role.' Such a view is echoed by Kugel and Parsons (1967) who report that mothers often accept an adolescent child 'as a peer, expecting him to carry the responsibilities of an adult.' One reason for this, according to Johnson and Clark (1984), is that parents with learning difficulties tend to lean on their children for emotional support and this 'emotional overinvestment is commonly associated with reverse dependency'. As they get older, it is claimed, the children too may become extremely protective of their parent 'to the point of managing the household at a young age' (Miller, 1994). Speaking as just such a child (Ciotti, 1989), Tammy Bachrach says she was seven when she first became aware that her mother was different. Not that it was a big deal: 'In the family it was just said that she was a slow learner.' As she got older, however, things began to change. At the age of ten, 'she began to notice a disconcerting role reversal. Instead of her going to her mother for advice, now, it seemed, her mother – who was by then divorced – was coming to her.'

O'Neill (1985) has provided the fullest examination so far of reverse dependency in families headed by a parent or parents with learning difficulties. She identifies five archetypal 'patterns of adaptation' among children brought up by such parents:

- *Rebellion* – where children rebel against their parents at an early age and, subsequently, against authority in general.
- *Pseudo-retardation* – where children take on 'the protective coloration of their cultural-familial retarded home environment'.
- *Other adjustment problems* – mainly concerning socialisation and control.
- *Parent's right hand* – where children 'take the parent's role very early in their lives'.
- *Normal adjustment* – meaning 'not merely the absence of obvious pathology, but effective striving towards socially approved personal goals'.

O'Neill argues that two of these characteristic adaptive outcomes – acting as a parent's right hand and rebellion – represent positive and negative sides respectively of the process of role reversal. In the former case, role reversal takes the form of caring for and protecting a parent and any younger children. In the latter case, it takes the form of the child disobeying and bossing the parent (and, later, other sources of authority). In both instances, O'Neill says, role reversal is precipitated by inadequate support for the parents. But whereas children who slot into the role of parent's right hand usually have some close adult outside the family with whom they can identify, their rebellious peers generally lack such a model.

Having established what is meant by the terms 'role reversal' and 'reverse dependency' in the literature on the subject, we now turn to the task of seeing if they find any echoes in the lived experience of the subjects in our study.

THROUGH THE LOOKING GLASS

What evidence was there of role reversal in the personal narratives of the now-adult children who told us their stories of growing up with a mother and/or father who had learning difficulties? People's perceptions of how well their parents had looked after them (and their brothers and sisters) and what domestic responsibilities, if any, they had assumed as children were topics that were discussed with all our informants. Here we use this material to assess how far the typical features of role reversal or reverse dependency highlighted in the literature were mirrored in people's childhood memories.

First, two points must be made about the fit between our methods and our mission. The notion of role reversal is usually held to apply in situations where the parent is disabled and the child is not. In fact, half of the children in our study were themselves disabled. Our approach has been to treat these people as a built-in comparison group giving us another angle of vision on parent-child relationships. Also, we did not interview all children in each family. Given that birth order, age and gender are factors known to affect children's involvement in caring for a disabled parent, it is possible that other siblings in the family, if not the person interviewed were, as Stafford (1992) puts it, 'supplementing the parents' parenting'. In this context, however, it is important to bear in mind the purpose of narrative research. Narrative is not a method suited to the testing of hypotheses. On the contrary, its strength lies precisely in slowing down the all-too-ready tendency to generalise by showing the full complexity of lives in the world. Our task here is simply to use people's stories to question whether the notion of role reversal is consonant with such complexity and captures the meanings people give to their own experience of growing up with a parent who has learning difficulties.

Starting with the literature reviewed at the beginning of this chapter, we have identified six 'narrative pointers' whose presence in our informants' accounts of their upbringing might be taken as a first indication of an underlying process of role reversal. The next step was to locate these narrative clues in the broader context of people's lives in order to establish if they properly justified such an interpretation.

Lost childhood

Any statements or comments conveying the impression that people had somehow missed out on their childhood were taken to suggest a prima facie link with the experience of young carers. As it turned out, none of the people who voiced such sentiments had carried any significant practical responsibilities in the home at any stage during their childhood or adolescence. Equally, in no case was this sense of loss associated by them with having a parent who had learning difficulties. Three main causes were linked with this way of thinking in people's personal narratives: the experience of abuse; chronic bullying and victimisation at school and in the community; and being taken into care. Veronica Stephenson is an example.

Veronica Stephenson

Veronica remembers moving house a lot as a child: Walnut Crescent, Walnut Place, Mablelee Road, Barnsthorpe Terrace, and more. . . .

> It were rough up Crackenly, and they used to pick on my mum with the way she was. She couldn't get any peace, she were terrified of going out. They never left her alone when she went to shop for something. She always came back upset.

The family would move, looking for a bit of respite, and for a time things would settle down, but eventually kids would start calling her mum names and picking on her, and the whole cycle would begin again. For all that, Veronica herself was not short of friends – 'We used to go round in groups and play out' – and up to the age of nine, she says, 'I were happy, I think I had a happy childhood. We were a right close family when we were little, we were really close.' Then, suddenly, her world fell apart.

> They accused me dad of hitting me and our Conrad with a puppy lead. They put us on twenty-eight-day care order and we were taken away. After them twenty-eight days we went back to court and we were kept in then.

Kept in for seven years. She was sixteen before the care order was finally lifted. Veronica hated it in the children's home.

> There were this woman, she were boss, and if you were naughty she used to make you play trees. You had to stand with your arms out, straight out side of you, and if you put them down she'd say put them up, you're not putting your arms down till I say so.

Veronica never blamed her parents for what happened: 'No, it were Social Services. I hated them.' She has no doubt that her life would have been different had she not been put in a children's home. Asked what she feels she missed, her response was immediate: 'Love and attention, my mum and dad.' 'When we went home for weekends, we saw family and it made me upset because I knew we'd have to go back. . . .' When Veronica did finally move back home at sixteen it was not easy to bridge the missing years. It 'felt strange', she says, 'You used to get used to routine of where you were living.' She had lost contact with her old friends and didn't see them anymore. Both she and her parents seemed to respond to their long separation by holding fast to each other. Veronica thought her parents needed looking after and 'felt as though I had to. . . . People kept saying "Mix with people". I didn't bother. I just looked after my mum and dad. I felt that, you know, I should be doing something, looking after them.' Her parents too, she felt, had 'got more stricter'; her dad, in particular, was 'too over-protective', insisting that she 'had to be in for half past nine'. Most of all, though, coming home left her with an abiding sense of sadness: 'I thought I'd lost summat . . . lost growing up.'

In contemporary society, childhood is commonly regarded as an age of innocence. Abuse, physical or sexual, is seen to represent an assault on innocence and hence a threat to the cultural meaning of childhood itself. There was a strong link between the experience of abuse and unhappy memories of childhood in the stories of our informants. Overwhelmingly, however, the perpetrators were people without learning difficulties (see chapter 4). The child did not necessarily have to be the victim for abuse to leave a mark. Philip Dawkins, who has learning difficulties like his mother, remembers only too well his father's tyrannical ways.

Philip Dawkins

Asked what he remembers about being a little boy, Philip replied straightaway, 'my dad come back from work and in a temper, and my dad hit Anne, that's my mum's name. Graham hit his wife.' This was no one-off incident. His father had quite a repertoire of cruel behaviour. Philip's mother used to play the piano, one bought for her by her parents, and he recalls how: 'My dad burnt that. My dad chopped it up, bonfire night, I remember it.' His father also chopped up Philip's junior desk, of which he was very proud. 'My dad not care about me. He never wanted me, he never wanted me to have those things. You'd think he would.' Philip was never really happy while he was around, and thinks he should have gone to prison. 'Graham keep hitting my mum all the time. And Graham say I won't do it again, he keep saying that. Mum got a lot of black eyes and bruises on the arm, Graham's done it.' Philip's parents finally divorced. 'He was no good, my dad,' Philip says, 'I hate him.'

Sometimes it was not the abuse itself but its consequences that marred people's childhood. Paula Clancy is one of eight children all with phenylketenuria, like their mother. Her father had been in the army.

Paula Clancy

About a year after the death of her mother, when she was ten, Paula and two of her sisters were raped by a neighbour. She was put on the 'at risk' register, and the man was convicted and imprisoned. Shortly after, her father was accused of 'touching me up' although she strenuously denies that he did any such thing, accusing her brother-in-law instead. She was placed in a children's home, where she had been lonely and homesick. Having always been 'a daddy's girl', she had missed her father badly, and when he died suddenly she was devastated. She remembers seeing his coffin, 'but to me he weren't dead'. She still visits the crematorium and would like to buy a plaque so that she has some-where to go and talk to him, but she can't afford one herself and her sisters aren't interested.

Parent's right hand

There were only four people in the study whose personal recollections of their own childhood and adolescence identified them as having played an important practical role in supporting a parent, looking after the family or maintaining the household. In three of these cases, the individuals concerned took on responsibilities, that would normally be considered beyond their years, in the absence from death or separation of one of their parents. Martin Riddick and Chris Sutton (see chapter 5) both took up the strain when their parents separated and their mothers, who had learning difficulties, were left to manage on their own. When Martin's mother moved to live closer to her own parents and sisters, the extra load that he'd been carrying was eased consider-ably, and when she found a new partner, Martin, by then in his late teens, was able to relinquish his role as 'the man of the house' – although, as he admits, 'At first, like, I were a bit wary because, this chap coming in, I think I felt a bit, like, having my nose pushed out of joint. I remember thinking, is he trying to, like, take over?' Chris Sutton also found that he had to do less when his parents got together again and remarried: 'It's a bit of a relief for him to come back into the family. It's like him taking over, giving me a rest point.' Maggie Lewis (see chapters 6 and 7) assumed primary responsibility in her teens, and in the absence of another adult in the household, for the care of her grandma, who had always been a mother-substitute, and a younger sister with learning difficulties. All three did what they did voluntarily, and none of them expressed any regrets about their lot. Maggie said

without hesitation, 'if I had my time to go back I'd do it all again".
Only Marie Summers, the fourth member of this group, was compelled
to take on caring duties against her will. Once again, the need came
about following the death of a parent, except in Marie's case the
survivor – her father – did not have learning difficulties.

Marie Summers

Marie is a quietly spoken, friendly young woman of twenty-seven who
initiates conversation once she feels at ease. Marie, an only child,
attended mainstream school until she was eleven, but was then moved
to a special school because, she says, 'I can't talk properly.'

Marie's parents are both now dead. Her mother, who had learning
difficulties, died when Marie was twelve years old. Her father was a
miner but had retired early after a pit accident in which he 'caught his leg
and had to limp every time'. She remembers him always with a walking
stick. He died when she was twenty-three. The years between were not
happy ones for Marie.

Returning from the chippy one day, her mother had fallen and injured
her leg: ' . . . blood come out and she cried and shouting and she need
some help. . . . There was all blood there . . . a right lot of blood. It was
right awful, right deep in her ankle.' The doctor called an ambulance,
'and I started screaming and shouting'. When her mother came home
from hospital, she was unable to walk and had to use a wheelchair. 'She
stayed downstairs. They fetched a bed and she sleep downstairs and
dad sleep upstairs. After that she had bad fits. She had bad fits and all
that, and then she died.'

Marie feels that the family could have done with some help after her
mother's accident, especially with shopping, housework and making the
fire. With both parents being disabled, the strain began to show. Marie
recalls how her 'dad kept shouting every time, making me do the jobs'.

After her mum died, Marie's father 'got another girlfriend in
Doncaster' and her life began to change. Whereas she used to feel over-
protected by her parents, now her father was sometimes away for a long
time and she was left alone in the house, often overnight: 'I used to stay
in house. Neighbours would come and see me. I used to feel awful, bit
scared, cried.' Her father had always done most of the domestic chores,
including most of the cooking. Marie says her mother used to go out
shopping, but otherwise it was mostly 'just telly, that's about all'. Now he
began making Marie stay at home to do the housework, and she missed
a lot of schooling.

After splitting up with his girlfriend, Marie's father took up with another woman and married her. Marie acquired a step-mother and three step-sisters, one of whom was still living with her mother. Together they all moved into a new house, taking Marie away from the elderly couple next door who had always kept an eye on her and to whom she felt close.

Marie felt as if she was losing her place in her father's affections: 'He didn't give me a lot of cuddles. He give them a lot of cuddles, just give her daughter a lot of cuddles.' Marie was made to do most of the washing, cooking, cleaning and ironing. Her step-mother, too, 'were cruel to me', beating her until she bruised. 'She went for kitchen knife, she got right mad to me. She hit me on my face, on my hands. She hit me on my leg and all that.' When Marie finally told her father: 'My dad got mad, he got mad. He went upstairs and just got right mad.' Soon afterwards he collapsed and died of a brain haemorrhage in the ambulance on his way to hospital.

Marie was left alone with her abusive step-mother and a step-sister who 'doesn't like me'. The exploitation and abuse, now unchecked, grew worse. Marie was prevented from going to college, and forced into domestic slavery. She was not allowed out, hit frequently and violently, often confined to her bedroom, and once denied food for a week as a punishment.

Marie was finally rescued by her old neighbours. One day, the phone rang. Her step-mother answered it and then

> flung telephone down and she got mad and she said, 'They know where I live.' They come and fetched me back, been looking for me. I started crying and all that. She swear at them. After that they took me to their house and I lived there until they got too old and now I live here for good.

In none of these cases was there a one-to-one relationship between the young person's caring and domestic responsibilities and their parent's learning difficulties. For Martin Riddick and Chris Sutton, the key factors that determined what they had to do for their mothers and siblings were their fathers' absence and the availability of external support. Maggie Lewis, out of a sense of duty, and Marie Summers, under duress, did their bit for people without learning difficulties. There is a sense, however, in which the notion of reverse dependency might be said to carry some weight. Some of the now-adult children with learning difficulties, who are usually cast in the role of dependents, were themselves looking after ill or ageing parents. Bonnie Craven (see chapter 4) has taken charge of the household now that her mother, severely depressed since her husband's death, has become something of a recluse, spending most of the day lying on her bed. Amos Ambler and his mother, both of whom have learning difficulties, lived with his maternal grandparents and when his grandma 'got bad on her legs', after his grandfather had died, they both looked after her together without any help from outside until she too passed away. Philip Dawkins is another case in point.

Philip Dawkins

Philip Dawkins and his sister, Jane, who also has learning difficulties, have managed the household and looked after their mother ever since she had a stroke which left her virtually bedbound. 'Mum don't walk any more, stroke's done it. She can talk, she can't move herself very well. She'll be sixty-two in July.' Aside from someone who comes in every day to 'wash my mum', Philip and Jane do all the everyday jobs in the home. Philip is responsible for the 'shopping every Thursday afternoon, shopping down Swillington' because he 'can do money'. He can't write very well but his 'sister can spell' so together they get by. Jane cooks the dinner, but Philip helps out with snacks like beans on toast. Jane usually does the washing and Philip tackles the ironing. They share the cleaning. This apparently neat division of labour doesn't always work out quite so smoothly in practice. 'Sometimes,' Philip says, 'Jane and I fall out at home.' At Christmas, their mum went into a nursing home and Jane and Philip joined her there for their Christmas dinner. Philip acknowledges that it's hard work looking after her, but he was glad to have her back home. He has voiced his concern that 'my mum might leave home for good soon. Mum says no.' A social worker visits but, Philip says, 'my mum doesn't like it.' She thinks he might be trying to steer her into a home and she doesn't want that. Philip has started to worry about Jane of late. She had an epileptic fit one night in bed while their mother was in the nursing home over Christmas. He had coped well, and called the doctor. Their mother 'had fits years ago' and Philip is now concerned that 'Jane could be like her mum now.' He's hoping she will 'grow out of it one day when she gets older.'

Rebellion

O'Neill (1985) cites rebellion as a form of role reversal linked directly to characteristics of households headed by a parent with learning difficulties – their frequent disorganisation and disruption – in which the child challenges parental authority in the home and is often then led to reject it outside. Rebellion of some kind was not an unusual feature in the backgrounds of people in our study. But their personal narratives show that it came about for a wider variety of reasons than O'Neill allows, making any simple link between rebellion and role reversal unreliable.

Bereavement was one of the factors associated with a rebellious phase in people's lives, especially when it led to the loss of a male authority figure or where parents became too wrapped up in their own grief to give their children the attention they needed. Adam Lloyd (see chapter 4) and his mother, who has learning difficulties, had lived with her parents throughout his early childhood: 'They says, "We'll help her fetch him up as her own," and they did.' When he was twelve, his grandfather died

> and that's when I started doing not going to school and all lot. They give me a week, says I'll give you a week's trial, took me back to school. I just kept saying I'm not going and I started getting a bit nasty with mum and grandma, like. I just kept thinking about my granddad and that and I didn't go and end up getting to go in a kid's home when I were twelve.

Maggie Lewis' story (see chapter 6) provides further evidence on the same lines. She too admits she 'went off rails when granddad died'. That Maggie always looked to her grandma as her mother warns against always treating the parent's learning difficulties as the first cause of rebellion in such families.

The break-up of the parents' relationship, like bereavement, is also a factor in children's rebellion, and for much the same reasons. It may entail domestic upheaval, grief over the loss of a parent, the loss of an authority figure, and a re-ordering of roles within the family. Martin Riddick admits that when his mum and dad divorced he thought of himself as being the 'man of house' and 'I probably felt I were getting a bit clever.' It was only when his aunties told him to get a grip of himself that 'I realised that I were getting bad and I thought, yes, you're not helping situation at all.'

Poverty also sparked off rebellion in young people. Missing out on holidays and school trips, birthday presents, treats and the latest toys at

Christmas all made them feel different. Unfashionable, hand-me-down clothes marked them out among their peers. Maggie Lewis only ever wore her sister's cast-offs. It was only when punk came along and 'you just wore everything scruffy' that she felt part of the crowd. At school or in the street being different meant being picked on, from teasing and cat-calling to bullying and ritual victimisation. Martin Riddick knew the score. When he started work he'd occasionally buy new clothes for his younger brother so as to prevent 'kids giving Keith a hard time at school'. 'I know what I went through,' he adds. Some fought back and got a name as troublemakers. Others dropped out of school, and were marked down as truants.

Sexual abuse was another factor tied in with rebellion. Veronica Stephenson admits that from about the age of fourteen she 'were always fighting' at school. She and her mum used to look after her elder brother's baby son on a Saturday, pushing him to the shops and round the market. Veronica's schoolmates 'used to say that were my child' and 'kept joking and saying that I were up stick to my brother'. These taunts were extra hard to bear because her older brother, some eight years her senior, who had spent all his childhood in care, had in fact been taking advantage of her during her weekend visits home from the children's unit. He'd first 'tried summat on' at their cousin's wedding when Veronica was thirteen and he, not then married, was twenty-two. Knowing that the jibes touched on a secret truth made Veronica deny them all the more vehemently: 'I got mad', she says. Sometimes 'I just snapped and used t' throw tables and chairs about.' Once, 'I got this lass and I were swinging her round by hair. I says, you ever say that again and you're going to be dead.' When a teacher slapped Veronica across the face for striking one of her tormentors, she 'cracked him back'. In the end, she was suspended from school six months before her sixteenth birthday and never returned.

Emotional overinvestment

According to Johnson and Clark (1984), parents with learning difficulties have a 'tendency to overinvest emotionally in their children.' When this happens, they say, 'the parent relies upon the child to provide needed emotional support'. It is not easy to tell when a parent has overstepped this boundary. For present purposes we have used three indicators of potential parental 'overinvestment' in children: *sexual abuse* as possibly an extreme manifestation of such a relationship 'where the role of substitute parent is taken to its logical conclusion' (Stafford,

1992); *leaving home at an early age* as a possible indication that children felt the need to break away in search of their own space; and *loneliness, social isolation and a lack of friends* as a possible sign that children have been tied too closely to their parents.

There was nothing in people's personal narratives to suggest that these indicators, even when present, provide evidence of reverse emotional dependency. None of the people in our study reported having been sexually abused by a parent with learning difficulties.

Although a large proportion of the men without learning difficulties left home while still quite young, the precipitating factor was invariably something other than their parent's disability. Keith Riddick moved out of the family home to live with his grandfather soon after his mother took up with a new partner:

> My mum and Ernie did row a lot and have quite violent arguments . . . a lot of shouting and sort of got aggressive. I thought I don't need this. I did have to sort of really get away, I just couldn't have carried on like that. It was obvious, I think, they needed each other, and once I realised that they weren't going to split up or anything like that, I thought I'm not going to live like this.

Chris Sutton left home and moved into a hostel for homeless people when he was seventeen because of all the rows he was having with his older sister. Mark Samuels went to live with a girlfriend when he was fifteen. No-one said or implied that a parent with learning difficulties had made too many emotional demands of them when they were younger, although the situation was not nearly so clear-cut in adulthood when several daughters in particular said they felt they were giving their mother with learning difficulties a lot of emotional support and getting none back when they needed it. For example, Veronica Stephenson:

> I still love her but I can't talk to her. She doesn't understand me when I talk to her. She doesn't want to listen to me. When I start talking she goes, she tells me what's gone on through day and what.

Maggie Lewis too doesn't feel she can talk to her mother, not 'talk to her properly'. Both she and her sister find they are always having 'to accept her apology all time . . . to forgive her' which they feel is the obverse of the usual parent-child relationship.

Finally, the personal narratives showed that lonely childhoods were mostly created by social exclusion and not by parents who relied on their children too much to allow them any independence or the freedom of play. It was segregated schooling, bullying, victimisation in the community (and the frequent efforts to escape by moving house), family breakdown and loss of contact with relatives that led to people having few friends as children. The majority of those who fell into this category also had learning difficulties themselves. To the extent that over-protectiveness was an issue for this group, it usually arose because their parents had learned from their own experience that the world is often a cruel place for people with learning difficulties, not because of any 'overinvestment' in their children. Luke Oliver is perhaps an exception to this general point, although in his case his parents' protectiveness stems from his own serious illness rather than from any emotional dependency on their part:

Luke Oliver

Luke Oliver is twenty years old and has learning difficulties. An only child, he lives with his mum and dad and pet dog in what used to be his grandparents' house. He has suffered persistent health problems since being a baby: first, with anaemia and eczema and then with recurrent blockage of the bowels. 'Since he were about three month old', his father says, 'he's been in and out of hospital nearly all his life.' At the age of sixteen he developed cancer of the stomach. His consultant decided that surgery would be too dangerous and he was given chemotherapy. He now attends the hospital once a year for a check-up.

Tall and slightly overweight, Luke has short brown hair and a wary disposition. He was wearing tracksuit trousers and a T-shirt. Having dropped out of further education college when he became seriously ill, he now spends most of his time at home with his parents, doing jigsaws, listening to his CDs, playing pool in the back bedroom or pursuing his interest in model railways.

Mrs Oliver has learning difficulties and at present she has a cleaning job for four hours a week, 'money in hand, keep yer gob shut'. Mr Oliver is a diabetic and used to work as a machine grinder until he was made redundant two years ago. Now he's on hand to keep Luke company when Mrs Oliver goes to work or does the shopping. They are both hugely protective of their son and took over the interview to talk about him.

Before his illness, Luke used to play outside in the street with his friends, kicking a football around and riding his bike. Now he has lost contact with the friends he made at school and has had no chance to make any new ones. His family – mum, dad, grandmother, uncle and aunt – are his only close associates. His parents are reluctant for him to attend college or a day centre because of his continuing bowel problems: his mother frankly admits, 'I don't like him going anywhere.' Part of their concern is that people 'might laugh at him and things like that. He has to carry his pads with him, don't he?'

The Olivers are making the most of their limited opportunities while Luke's tumour is in remission. As Mrs Oliver said, 'Still on your mind, you never forget it, no chance. You don't know, you just live day to day, don't we? You don't know.'

Care of siblings

If parents really do abdicate their role in favour of a son or daughter it might also be expected that the child who steps into their shoes will assume a parenting role in respect of any younger brothers and sisters and, Little Dorrit fashion, become a mother or father to the rest of the family. Seven of the thirty people in our study were only children. It was not always easy to determine exactly how many brothers and sisters the remainder had or how many children had been living in the household with the informant as a child. The picture was confused by a changing cast of half-brothers and sisters, family break-up and reconstitution, children moving into and out of care or backwards and forwards between different family members, and the number of one-time multiple households. Equally, it was not possible to define any fixed standards for judging whether anyone was acting more like a parent to their siblings than a brother or sister. Any such judgement must be influenced by a wide range of considerations including family size, birth order and spacing, family composition, the age of the children, the parents' employment and so on. Older children in large families with a single working parent would normally be expected to play a bigger part in caring for younger brothers and sisters than their counterparts in smaller, two-parent families. Cutting through these problems, and again referring back to the narrative content of people's stories, the only safe conclusion seems to be that, where parents' parenting needed supplementing, it was more likely to be grandparents, and sometimes an aunt or uncle, who took on the responsibility than a son or daughter. Sixteen – over half – of the people in the study either lived with or close to their grandparents as a child. Tracy Talbot illustrates the point.

Tracey Talbot

Tracey Talbot is the eldest of five children. She is twenty-five years old and lives with her husband, Cliff, and their three small children in a reno-vated, three-bedroom semi on a large council estate. Tracey's parents live about a mile away. Her mother is partially sighted, and has suffered from thrombosis since her second child, Dennis, was born. Tracey's father has learning difficulties, and has lost most of the use of one arm which he shattered in a fall some years ago. Both parents had attended special school. Tracey's two brothers and two sisters still live at home with their parents. Her sisters, Rita (thirteen) and Kim (eleven), are still at school, and her brothers, one of whom, Dennis, has learning difficulties, are unemployed. Both Dennis (twenty-four) and his younger brother, Mark (eighteen), have tried living in their own flats but the bills and the loneliness drove them back home.

As a child, Tracey lived for long spells with her maternal grandpar-ents, after Dennis was born, because her mother had to spend so much time in hospital: 'We were on and off with my grandma and granddad. She practically brought us up all time.' Her father was working as a window cleaner in his own father's firm and he too stayed with them.

Their first house had been bought for them by Tracey's mother's parents and was situated across the road from their own: 'we were always backwards and forwards to my nan's.' Tracey has never had much to do with her grandparents on her father's side: 'They like my dad's brother's kids better than such as us. I don't know why, but that's how it's always been.'

Tracey never went short of anything as a child. 'I got practically everything I wanted', she says. 'I were first, so I got everything. I even had one of them little fur coats with little muffs on.' She looks back on her childhood as a happy time:

> I can always remember going out, trips and stuff with my grandma and granddad, and my mam and dad. Used to have a good time and used to go out, like while my mum and nan-nan did dinner, like Sundays, granddad and my dad'd take us to a park or summat, or somewhere in the country. We used to go all o'er. And odd weekends we used to go away for a day or summat, you know what I mean, Skeggy or Cleethorpes or summat.

'I can always remember me and our Dennis always had loads of fun.' They used to stick up for each other. She remembers when Dennis once punched the dentist who was attending to her teeth because 'he thought they were hurting me.' And she, in turn, 'stuck up for him when people's been taking michael out of him and calling him nasty names and stuff, laughing at him. I hate it, to see anybody doing that to him.' Tracey has never really felt she had to look after her younger brother and sisters. She says:

> It's funny to see Rita, Kim and Mark now, like to how me and Dennis were when we were little. It's completely different. They're, like, out of control, but when me and Dennis were little we weren't nowt like that. We were like angels compared to them.

The telling difference, she thinks, is that 'they haven't had my nan-nan and granddad to look after them like we had.' Her grandparents 'kept you in order'. Indeed, as she got older she found

> they were strangling you, sort of thing. You couldn't go here, you couldn't go there, you'd got to be in for this time, that time. They'd pick you up from school no matter whether you wanted to be picked up or not. My mum's easier going, a lot easier.

When Tracey thinks back to who used to do the jobs in the house, she says, 'I suppose it was me and my mum'. In fact, Tracey used to do the 'usual things like helping her to tidy up, keep your rooms and that tidy, wash up.' It was her mum who did the bulk of the housework, and the cooking, washing and ironing. Tracey concedes that it was only, 'If you were desperate for summat you did it yourself.' She doubts if her parents found it any harder to manage when she married and set up her own home; the only difference her going made, she suspects, is that 'there were more room for everybody else.' Tracey still sees her mum every day. 'I go up a lot', she says, 'Help my mum tidy up when she needs it and she can't get others to do it. If I want owt doing she'll come and help me, or if she wants something I go and help her.' Every weekend her youngest son goes to stay with her parents and her middle lad goes to her husband's mum's, as they have done since they were a few weeks old. 'I suppose', she says, 'they've been brought up with their nan-nans and granddads anyway'; just as it was 'My mum's mum and dad who looked after us.' Tracey thinks she has a close relationship with her mum. She's not so sure about her dad. 'Your mum's always there for you anywhere.'

For Keith Riddick, it was his aunties – his mother's sisters – who watched over him and his brothers, and when his father left home to live with another woman 'the women took over really, they did.' It was his aunties who kept the boys in order, made sure they had clothes for school, sorted out their mum's social security, looked after them when their mum was ill:

> Mum did care for us. She wasn't, you know, the brightest person. But no, she did care for us best as she could, you know, but it were just in her own way. We seemed to sort of cope fairly well on us own but we did have that reassurance of aunties being there. It was, like, a loving family, they did really pull for each other. My mum being the youngest of the girls, I think they were very protective of her.

Negative outcomes

It has been argued that young caring interferes with the normal processes of child development and may lead to detrimental effects in later life. There were too few people in our study who had taken on any serious caring responsibilities as children to provide a proper test of this claim. However, two general points are worth making.

People who look for problems will invariably find them. That is why the police see crime everywhere and social workers see only dysfunctional families. People with learning difficulties are almost always described in terms of their limitations rather than their strengths, their deficits rather than their capacities, what they can't do rather than what they can do. There is a similar bias in the literature on young caring which emphasises the negative outcomes and skirts over any positive benefits. Yet there has been no research so far that has followed young carers into adulthood in order to establish how they look back on their earlier experience in the context of their later lives. None of the people in our study who had taken on caring responsibilities as children or young people looked back with any sense of loss or resentment. Indeed, if anything their attitude was the opposite. When Keith Riddick was eighteen his mum took up with a new partner and he left home to live with his granddad. His granddad

> was getting on (and) he did suffer a lot with, I suppose to quite a degree, with dementia. It was hard work actually. You didn't know what state the house was in when you got back in, he used to leave gas on and he was very forgetful, or doors open, go out, leave the doors unlocked. It was almost like looking after a child, I did a helluva lot there. I think it was my grandfather that probably learnt me to appreciate having to do your own thing and to depend on yourself: not a skill from him but because of him. It's probably given

me that independence, made me stronger, it's that responsibility really.

Another cautionary note is sounded by the stories of the people in our study: it is too easy to assume a direct link between parental disability and negative child outcomes. A lot of research is about simplifying things to the point at which generalisation is possible. The narrative approach endeavours to face up to the complexity of human experience even if it often fails in the goal of 'capturing the totality, the process and the meaning.' (Faraday and Plummer, 1979). Too much research into young carers has simply assumed that parental disability constitutes the independent variable in the analysis of outcomes. Narrative accounts of people's real-life experience underline Parker and Olsen's (1995b) point that 'the causality is difficult to pin down'. Material deprivation, social exclusion, discrimination, victimisation and the inadequacies of the support services, ranging from resource starvation through to full-scale system abuse (see chapter 9), play a part in shaping disabled people's parenting. From this point of view, disabled parenting is just as much a social creation as disability itself.

CONCLUSION

Role reversal or reverse dependency are not concepts that found any resonance in the memories or experience of the now-adult children in our study. They simply do not fit their perceptions of the relationship they had with their parents.

The first rule of narrative research is to listen. In fact, following Studs Terkel's advice, it is also the second, and the third, and the fourth: 'Listen . . . listen . . . listen . . . listen' (Parker, 1996). If, having listened, we then proceed to theorise over people's voices, forcing their lives into boxes and categories that do not relate to their experience or match their view of the world, there is little reason for collecting their stories in the first place. On this basis, we must conclude that the upside down family is a myth.

Chapter 9

System abuse and the limits of advocacy

Eric Burgess was thirteen when his parents separated. In the next few years he and his mother moved address nine times, sometimes sleeping in condemned properties, once in an outside toilet. They finally settled in a small council house close to where Emily's family lived.

It was some time before Eric and Emily got to know each other. They had attended different schools as Emily, who has learning difficulties, had been bussed to a special school outside the area. When both were in their early twenties, they started going out together.

Emily had been going with Eric for a year when she discovered she was pregnant. In the face of opposition from both their mothers, they decided to get married. Emily's mother wanted her to have an abortion. Emily herself was in no doubt that she wanted to keep the baby. She was five months pregnant when they married. After the wedding, they moved into her mother's two-up and two-down terraced council house.

A son, Jack, was born and, two years later, a daughter, Annie. By now there were ten people living in the house: Emily's mother, Emily and Eric and their two children, Emily's brother, and Emily's divorced sister with her three children. In some ways this arrangement suited Emily and Eric well. With her mother and sister around, there was always help available for Emily during the day until Eric came home from work. It was six years before they finally acquired a home of their own, and within a couple of weeks Eric's mother had moved in to live with them. She did the cleaning, made the meals, helped with the children and kept Emily company. In 1982, Emily, unexpectedly pregnant again, had another son, Simon. Five years later Eric's mother died and their troubles began.

Until Emily was left to cope on her own, Eric had not realised the full extent of her limitations. Always having lived in a household where support was on hand, he had not grasped that she could not manage a domestic routine. The house began to show signs of neglect. Meals were a hit-or-miss affair, rubbish accumulated, and Eric had to take over the ironing and washing because Emily could not understand the dials.

Eric took his mother's death very hard and slipped into a severe depression. He thought seriously about splitting up the family. Emily and the children would go back to her mother and he would go it alone. He found it more and more difficult to work when all the time he was fretting about what was happening at home. On the other hand, if he took time off to help out, he worried about losing his job. In the end he was made redundant.

It was round about this time that their eldest boy, Jack, began to mix with the wrong crowd. He was found by police breaking into houses and damaging property, and was fortunate to be let off with a formal caution. Annie too began to truant from school. She was going about with a group of girls who were messing in petty thieving. Occasionally she'd go missing for a day or two at a time. Her dad began to suspect something altogether more sinister was amiss when she started vandalising her own bedroom – making holes in the walls, writing on the wallpaper – and wetting her bed at night. There was talk about a paedophile ring on the estate.

Fearing for his daughter, Eric started to keep her at home where he knew she was safe. Until the police nailed the abusers, he reasoned, it was up to him to protect her as best he could. Annie was kept out of school month after month, until finally the education authorities woke up to her absence. When she was fifteen the police accused her of theft; Annie was taken into care and put in a children's home. Eric and Emily, apparently unable to save their daughter from the tow of events pulling her under, began to question their own fitness as parents.

Annie had been in the children's home for just a few weeks when I first called at their house. The Burgesses had agreed to take part in an interview study of families headed by a parent or parents with learning difficulties. Three interview sessions were planned with each family. As I pulled up outside and braced myself for the introductions to come it never crossed my mind that I might still be tied up with the family six years later.

THE BURGESS FAMILY: A RESEARCH DIARY

September 1991

My first visit to the family. Their living room is warm and cosy. Council workmen are in the street re-painting the houses. Eric makes us all a coffee.

Emily tells me that she is attending college where she does cooking and learns about being healthy. Her social worker had got her onto the course.

Eric has recently checked out their benefits with a claimant adviser and discovered that Emily is entitled to Severe Disability Allowance. This extra cash, along with money saved from Eric giving up smoking, has enabled them to start running a car and they are enjoying regular trips out into the countryside. Eric says he's also eligible for Attendance Allowance but he'd rather have a job and hasn't done anything about claiming it yet.

Eric talks about Annie. He feels the police and social services have never taken his fears seriously.

> I mean, she's told me that some chaps in a red Range Rover used to pick them up from down town. . . . I started keeping a diary for last couple of years. Had all these different dates when different people have called for her.

They give me their ex-directory phone number, and I give them my home number in return.

October 1991

Emily is on her own. She is going on a day trip to Blackpool soon with Simon, Annie and some social workers. Annie is due for an assessment and then there will be a review: they are hoping she will be coming home after her next birthday. Her two brothers are missing her. Emily rings her every day.

Emily says she has no friends in the neighbourhood, but she's made some at college and has always been close to her family. She talks briefly about the support worker who helps with the shopping.

Emily phones a couple of times during the next fortnight. Annie's review has been postponed because the social worker was ill, but she'd spent the night at home after their trip to Blackpool. They are expecting a delivery of furniture organised by their social worker.

The next time I visit, Emily's support worker is there. Emily calls her 'mother'. Eric explains her job is 'to try and give Emily some sort of routine, like help her to do things.' She's been coming for a couple of months, two hours twice a week, ever since Annie went into the children's home. It soon becomes clear why the place is so neat. Her parting comment to Emily is, 'Get Simon to put his rubbish away in that cupboard or I'll put you in it.' Eric gets told in equally strong terms to wash the windows outside.

Annie is still not back in school and there's talk of her going to live with a foster family. Eric and Emily see her as much as they can. 'We have two access days a week, Wednesdays and Sundays, and unlimited talking on the phone.' When they took her back the other day after a trip out, they noticed that all the downstairs windows of the children's home had been smashed and were now boarded up. It left them feeling anxious that she might be more vulnerable in care than at home.

A week later Emily phones to say the review will take place in six days time. Annie says she still loves them very much.

November 1991

Annie's review has been and gone. She'd done a bunk and missed the proceedings. She was found eventually at a friend's house. Annie had visited the prospective foster family twice, but didn't want to go.

Most of the people at the review had been standing in for the main participants who were otherwise engaged. A social worker had told them that the police were trying to gather as much evidence as possible about the paedophile ring before making an arrest. Eric has once again been left doubting his role as a father. 'You feel like they're telling you you're inadequate as a parent.' He fears that now 'Annie's gone into care it won't be long before they're taking Simon.'

Emily phones to ask for my address as she wants to send me a Christmas card. Her social worker is getting them a new cooker, and an eiderdown and pillows for their bed. They've bought Annie a 50cc moped for her birthday in January.

December 1991

Their phone has been cut off. Emily has been ringing Annie in the children's home every day and when the bill came through it was over a hundred pounds. They couldn't pay. Contacting Annie is now a problem as she is often out when they phone from a call box and she can't ring them back.

Emily has received some credits for work done at college. She is hoping to make a cake for Annie's sixteenth birthday in the cooking sessions. At present her class is busy baking mince pies and a chocolate log for Christmas.

Eric has become depressed by events in the family and has taken himself off his Employment Training Scheme. Consequently his income support has been temporarily stopped along with the automatic rent payments. With Christmas approaching, he is facing a financial crisis as bills mount up for the rent and the poll tax. They are thinking of moving out of the area because of what has happened to Annie, although they've had their name down for re-housing since 1987 with the idea of moving back nearer to Emily's mother.

January 1992

The family owe £130 for rent. Things were a bit tense over Christmas as Eric and Emily were unable to buy anything. They had been awarded a temporary payment but Emily had slipped the crossed giro into her handbag and Eric had found it too late to cash it before the holidays. The social worker has managed to get them a grant for a cooker and some new lino. She'd also bought the family a few little presents for Christmas, as had their support worker.

Annie had spent Christmas with them, and is going to be allowed home every Saturday, although Eric is unhappy about her coming back into the neighbourhood. 'I feel that things could just start again from where we left off.' Social services have told them that the reason she'd been skipping school was because friends were bullying her into visiting the man's house where the sexual offences had occurred – as Eric had told them all along. Annie is currently receiving just two days schooling a week at an adolescent unit. It's on the cards that she'll return home after her sixteenth birthday in January.

On Sunday they had all travelled to the seaside in their car. Eric feels such weekend trips give them a break from the pressures in their lives.

Emily phones a couple of times at the end of January to ask when I'll be calling again. When I drop by she's out at college, but Eric is at home. He tells me that Annie had been taken to the local police station by a member of staff from the children's home and given a formal caution about the alleged theft. Eric and Emily had only found out when Annie told them afterwards.

March 1992

Eric and Emily have received a report on Annie's progress. It's the first they have been sent, although they have attended four case conferences altogether. They have no idea what has been written in the previous reports. Eric feels that 'if someone asked me why she's in children's home, I can't give a direct explanation.'

Annie has been in the children's home for seven months now. The fostering arrangement had been unsuccessful and a supported lodging scheme has now been mooted as a possibility. Eric feels she might be at risk in this scheme because of its proximity to where the sexual offences took place. He has agreed reluctantly to let her give it a try if she wants. Emily and Eric have been told by their social worker that the man Annie accused of molesting her has been arrested. Eric still believes he is only the front for a paedophile ring.

Annie's education is still limited to two days a week at the adolescent unit. Recently, staff have been dropping her off at the unit but she has been taking herself to the local leisure centre. They are now trying to get her on a youth training scheme.

Eric and Emily talk about recent happenings at the children's home. Two young people had overdosed on paracetamol and another young lad had smashed the place up. They have seen changes in Annie too. 'She's got a bit more aggressive, she's a bit more demanding than she used to be. Used to be quiet and placid.' Her enuresis problem is still troubling her. Eric thinks he knows the cause: 'I'm sure it's stress, nerves related problem, than a physical problem.' She has found herself a boyfriend, Ricky, who lives at the home.

Eric has been awarded Attendance Allowance for Emily. 'It'll put me back in arrears again until it's sorted out – having to come off income support.'

He talks about their support worker.

> She'll not let you get away with owt, not let you slack. She's got a list of different things to do for days of week, and what should be done on a certain day, and she'll tick you off if they're not done.

She uses the promise of treats to make Simon do as she wants. 'She'll say, "I'll not take you swimming if you don't do that." '

April–May 1992

Annie is at home and working on an ET scheme. A review is planned for 28 May to see if she can stop at home permanently. She is still seeing her boyfriend Ricky from the children's home, and he comes round most evenings.

Jack has found himself a job as a car mechanic. He has been fined £150 with six penalty points for driving his van without MOT and insurance. The van has since been stolen.

Eric and Emily are hoping to move house on medical grounds now they are receiving Attendance Allowance. Even so, Eric has redecorated the kitchen and stripped the lounge ready for papering.

June 1992

Annie has finally been discharged from the children's home, although she still visits people there. Simon is causing some upset at home and has smashed the banister rail in half.

Eric is not sure he can be bothered to finish the decorating. Their social worker has painted the ceiling. Eric says she did it to motivate him: 'She knows I can't sit and look at it now like this, got to finish it off. Crafty move.' He still feels frustrated and angry about what has happened to Annie, so much so that he kicked a hole in the living room door. He has since patched it up.

Jack's moped has been taken from their garden shed and set on fire by a group of lads. He hasn't been able to claim anything on insurance because the excess on his policy exceeded the bike's value. Jack and Eric have since been to the motor auctions and bought Jack a car. Jack used to be bullied a lot at school and left six months early because he couldn't take any more. Local youths have threatened to steal Eric's car in the past: 'I said, I'll know where to come if it does. Next minute door'd been peed on.'

July–August 1992

Although Annie is now living at home, she occasionally stops at her boyfriend's flat overnight. Her review has gone according to plan and the next one is arranged for January.

Emily phones to say they are moving house very soon. Apparently they had received a letter asking them to call in at the Area Housing Office that same day. They were made an offer of a transfer there and then, given until the afternoon to accept, and four days in which to move. They had decided to sign. She gives me their new address.

September 1992

I call at their new house, but Emily has given me the wrong address. I try their old house but the neighbours don't know where they have gone. The Housing Department cannot tell me for reasons of confidentiality. I go in search of their social worker to find out where they are. It's a week before I finally track them down.

Eric and Emily seem much more buoyant and give me a guided tour of the house and garden. Their new house is set at the end of a cul-de-sac next to a grassy recreational area. The drains are blocked with rubbish and smell quite badly but Eric and Jack have made a start on clearing the garden.

A public footpath runs by the side of the house giving a much-used short cut to the shops and pub. Eric suspects that rubbish might get thrown into their garden. There is no central heating in the house and most of the windows have been replaced at some time. Eric is pleased with new net curtains he has bought for the front window.

They have found out that the house has been unoccupied for the past eighteen months and are wondering why they were rushed into accepting the transfer. Although they had wanted to move, they had not liked being pressured into making a quick decision. On balance, though, Eric feels happier being away from those 'bad influences' that had smitten the family in their previous home. They see themselves as having the opportunity to make a fresh start.

The council has given them a removal grant of £360 towards new decorations but they have had to use some of the money to live on until their benefits are sorted out. Their social worker has helped them complete an application for new carpets, and Emily's sister has offered them her old three-piece suite.

Eric can't afford to MOT or road tax his vehicle, but Jack's car is roadworthy again and, having lost his job, he spends his time running errands, ferrying his mum back and forth to her college classes and helping his dad in the garden. Eric has resigned himself to not working again now that he receives Attendance Allowance. He says at least he'll have more time for his family and for decorating. Simon has slotted into his new school and made friends with the young lad next door. Annie is still with Ricky and hoping to move out soon into her own place.

They've been told that their social worker will be changed as they now come under a different local team. They don't know what is happening about their family support worker.

Eric has noticed the police on the estate in the early hours of the morning talking to groups of youths.

October 1992

Both their old support worker and social worker have paid them a visit. No decision has yet been made about allocating them a new social worker, but they will not be getting a new family support worker. The Housing Department has billed them £77.66 for 'dismantling and clearing tenant's timber hut and removing a small amount of rubbish' from the garden of their previous tenancy. They'd had to move out in such a rush there'd been no time to shift the shed.

The living room has been painted and a new pink carpet lays wrapped ready for fitting, a present from Emily's mum. Their old settee and chairs look shabby in these fresh surroundings and they are still awaiting the suite promised by Emily's sister. They are watching an old black-and-white TV which their social worker had once given them.

Emily has been awarded three credits for Level One English. She can now write her name on her child benefit book.

Annie has a job at some stables. She hasn't made any new friends in the neighbourhood but Eric doesn't think she is bothering with the old ones who had led her into trouble. The neighbours have been talking about the amount of crime that goes on in the area to finance drugs. 'There's a group of local youths that are undesirable. I've seen them coming across our back with stolen property. So we've kept us selves to us selves here.' Eric remains unsure about whether they have made the right move: 'I still have my apprehensive moments.'

As I leave I see that Eric has fitted a heavy brass lock to the front door.

December 1992

A burnt-out car sits in the road opposite their house and I feel uneasy as I knock on the door. This is my last scheduled visit as part of the research study that was the reason for my first contacting them. Inside, Eric and Emily are feeling the cold. They'd had central heating in their old house and they miss it now.

The harassment has become much worse since my last visit. 'We've had us window put through at back . . . with a piece of concrete.' Eric had put his hand up to protect his face and been badly cut.

> It were after car got afire. It went quiet for a bit because they were all at pub drinking. You could hear them shouting and ranting and they come all way down road. They were on corner there, at side of flats, drinking, and I just went out and said, can you keep your noise down, and they said, 'Come on let's get him'. So I dashed in and got spade, chased them back a bit, but they were just too many for me and then that's how window got broke.

The window had been replaced, but another one has been broken since. Eric says, 'You see, they're feeling you out.'

Eric and Emily have begun to feel unsafe and have taken the electric kettle and tea things into the living room away from the kitchen window. The flats behind have also been set on fire. Emily is frightened and Eric fears for the safety of the whole family. He's put their name down for a transfer or mutual exchange. 'There's about three moved off since we've moved on.' Their neighbour is also wanting to move away after twenty-two years on the estate. 'She said it's got worse over last two or three year.'

Emily has seen her old social worker. 'She says she feels sorry for us, she helped us to get to here.' They've still not heard if they've been allocated a new one.

Annie has been summoned to give evidence in court about her sexual exploitation. Eric says, 'I've got to go with her. I don't want her to get back in with them again. That was one of reasons for moving.'

As I make my goodbyes, I feel it is a depressing end to our long contact and to a relationship that has developed way beyond the compass of my study. I am unable to say anything to give them cheer. I say we can stay in touch if they like, although I shan't be calling as I have been doing any more.

Two weeks later Emily phones to tell me her sister's husband has died.

January–March 1993

Emily phones every few weeks to keep me up to date with her news. They are still hoping to move and appear to think their old social worker is sorting something out for them. They've started packing their stuff in anticipation. Eric has taken to meeting Emily from college and then both of them go into town because they are too frightened to stay in the house.

In the middle of March, Emily phones from hospital to tell me that Annie has just given birth to a baby boy, Billy. The news comes as a shock, but Emily sounds thrilled. Evidently, Annie had said nothing until her waters broke. With being quite plump, and wearing baggy clothes, she had managed to keep her pregnancy secret. Emily had never even suspected, although Eric says the thought had crossed his mind. Annie and baby Billy are going to live with Ricky's mother.

April 1993

An Easter card comes through the post from Emily, and on Easter Monday both of them phone just to say hello.

I receive a telephone call from an educational psychologist. Simon is due to be assessed because his parents are keeping him away from school. Eric had given him my name as someone who knew a lot about the family and what they had been through. I agree to write a summary of the family's difficulties over the time I have known them, but only with Eric and Emily's express permission. He says he'll contact me again later.

I call at Emily and Eric's and relate my conversation with the psychologist. They would like me to write and I promise to let them see my statement. *(In the event, I never hear from the psychologist again.)*

Baby Billy is now in care. The boyfriend of Ricky's mother's had returned and didn't want her to have the baby. Annie and Ricky are looking for a flat of their own.

May–July 1993

Emily phones several times. Annie and Billy are going into a mother and baby unit until December. Eric and Emily are hoping to get a bigger house so that the two of them can move in with them.

August 1993

Annie is back living with Ricky. Billy has been placed with foster parents. Emily is desperate to move. She says they need help and still have no social worker almost a year after their move. I ask for her permission to phone social services on their behalf.

It takes me two days to track down someone who can tell me why the Burgesses have not been re-allocated a social worker. (Goodness knows how anyone gets through from a public phone box.) I am told that as Emily comes under the Disability Section it could take months and months. I point out that until they get a new social worker they can't be referred for a family support worker either. I am also informed that Annie's social worker would not want to assist in re-housing the Burgesses as she does not think it is in the baby's interests for him to live with his mother's parents.

I call to see Emily and Eric. They tell me that Annie cannot have Billy living with her whilst she is with Ricky because he is a Schedule 1 offender. Billy may be permanently fostered.

September–December 1993

Emily continues to keep me in touch with what is going on. Annie is thinking of leaving Ricky because she wants to keep Billy. There'd been talk of him being adopted. Annie is hoping to go back to the mother and baby unit. Emily and Eric are only able to see Billy once a fortnight at Emily's sister's. Emily still wants Annie and the baby to live with them, but only if they move from their present house.

Simon is still not attending school because the other kids 'are tormenting him'.

January–May 1994

Annie is back living with Ricky's mother who has fostered Billy. Eric's car has been vandalised and their house has been burgled. Emily has been to see her doctor for a letter supporting their application for re-housing on health grounds.

November 1994

I call to see Emily and Eric as there has been no word from them for a long time.

Since fostering Billy his paternal grandmother has had a nervous breakdown. Eric says that social services are 'pushing for adoption'.

They are worried about Simon who has not been attending senior school and they don't know how to get him to go. I ask their permission to contact the Education Department about the situation. When I ring the Educational Welfare Officer, she says she has been twice to the house to see Simon in the past, but somehow he seems to have fallen between the cracks. She says he should be getting extra tuition at school and possibly transport to get him there. I explain that extra support is needed to mobilise the family in order to get Simon to that stage, and point out that social services have withdrawn the support they used to provide. She agrees to pay them another visit.

A meeting is fixed a week later at Eric and Emily's house, and I go along to give them moral support. Simon is present. All three agree to the Education Welfare Officer calling in a morning and walking with Simon to school.

My work elsewhere prevented any further visits for over a year, although Emily continued to phone periodically. Annie spent a few months living in a hostel for home-less women. The man charged with sexual offences against her was convicted and sent to prison. Simon started to attend school but, after Christmas, he slipped back into his old habit of going to bed late and not getting up in the morning. Early in 1995, his school was burnt to the ground in an arson attack and, though temporary classrooms were in place quickly, he never went back. Jack found himself a job in January and, with him off the dole, Emily and Eric had to start paying rent. Jack gave them nothing for his keep and arrears accumulated fast. Victimisation of the family continued unabated. Paint stripper had been poured over their cars, their garden was used as a rubbish tip by other residents, guttering and waste pipes had been wrenched off, they'd had to board up some windows, gangs of kids tormented them in the street chanting and name-calling, and they had been burgled twice more. They were unable to afford household insurance and had to carry the losses them-selves. The family remained fearful of staying in the house and continued to visit the local shopping mall nearly every day, but leaving the house empty made it an easy target for vandals and thieves and eating out was expensive. Emily's health had deteriorated. She was having trouble swallowing solid foods and had lost a lot of weight. In July, almost three years after their move, they received a letter from the Social Services Disability Section informing them that Emily would not be allocated a social worker and that her file had been closed: she would have to call in at the office four miles away to see a duty officer if she needed help. Both Eric and Emily were missing little Billy. Now that he was fostered out of the family they were unsure about their rights concerning contact. Annie felt that if her parents had remained in their old house she and Billy would have moved in with them. There was no way she could contemplate doing that now because of the violence directed against the family and the very real danger from flying glass and stones.

Late in 1995, I began an action research project aimed at developing an advocacy support network for parents with learning difficulties and their partners. The Burgess family agreed to join the project and, in January 1996, I became their advocate. Once again I started to keep a research diary recording everything that passed between us. My first task was to get them to list their priorities for the future. Eric and Emily were quite clear in their own minds about what they wanted: to move off the estate and to get Simon back into school.

February 1996

Another pane of glass has been smashed in the front window. The house is now almost completely boarded up so that lights have to be kept on during the day. Eric has saved all the missiles for evidence and stacked them into a small wall in the front room. The council will undertake repairs free of charge only when a crime number has been issued, but Eric is fed up with reporting the breakages to the police. In any case, they feel safer behind their shutters.

Emily is waiting for a hospital appointment to see a specialist. A barium x-ray has confirmed that her eating difficulties have been caused by a narrowing of the gullet.

They have been told that a place is now available for Simon at special school. He could be collected by the same taxi that calls for a neighbour's child. No-one from Education has been to see the family despite the recommendation in Simon's statement that 'the most important consideration would be to get someone to make a relationship with both him and his parents'. Simon is still wetting his bed.

Annie has been thrown out of her hostel for upsetting another resident and is back living with her parents. She is waiting for her own flat. Eric confides that hearing the evidence in court about what Annie went through has 'prevented me and Emily from having any further sexual enjoyment in marriage'.

Eric has collected a parking ticket – £20 rising to £30 if not paid within seven days. He has already been summoned to appear before the Magistrates' Court in March for failing to keep up with payments of £3 a week on an earlier fine of £330 he received for twice being caught without road tax. His car is currently insured, but he still has no tax, a bald tyre, and the MOT runs out soon. It's only a matter of time before he's caught again. They have also just received their council tax demand for £153.

Eric and Emily have been down to the Area Housing Office to ask about moving. They were told that their case would not be considered until their rent arrears were cleared, unless they were prepared to accept a transfer to a hard-to-let property on the same estate. I suggest that we write to Housing presenting all the reasons why they have to move off the estate.

Their next door neighbour is in hospital after trying to commit suicide. Mud has been thrown at their boarded-up windows.

March 1996

They have been burgled again. Emily's handbag and purse were taken. Another window has been smashed while they were out, and their car windscreen broken. A neighbour whose car was also damaged reported the incident. When the policewoman came round she asked Eric and Emily, 'What have you done to upset them?', as if it was their fault. Three cars have been burned out on the recreation area behind their house in the past week.

Annie has moved into her own flat, but Eric says she and Ricky still pop home 'when their money runs out'.

We make a chart of their cash flow to see how best to deal with their mounting debts. They have incurred bank charges of £25 for overdrawing by ten pounds on their current account. We talk about disposing of their car and possibly borrowing from the Social Fund to pay off their debts. Eric thinks they could meet the repayments from their benefit monies. He recognises that if he continues to keep the car on the road illegally he might end up in prison. But giving it up means they will be trapped on the estate. He had not attended when his case came up before the Magistrates' Court and is now two payments in arrears on his fine.

April 1996

Annie has agreed to Billy's adoption although she hasn't yet signed the form. She still wishes she'd been given the chance to look after him. She is concerned about her father's debts. He has told her he would rather go to prison than carry on as they are. Prison, he says, would provide an escape from stresses that are becoming unbearable. Annie has a new boyfriend, Ben.

Seemingly Eric sent a copy of the letter we had written to Housing to the police. An officer phones me having been to see Eric and Emily. He feels they might stand a better chance of a new house if 'they made their house and themselves look better'. He agrees that victimisation is a police matter but says they cannot do anything unless Eric and Emily are prepared to make a statement naming the culprits. He acknowledges that first-time offenders are only likely to get a verbal warning.

Eric suspects that Housing might not know Emily is registered as disabled. He had assumed that this information would have been forwarded in their file by their previous Area Housing Office. He also thinks that Housing still assumes that Jack is working because he is not signing on. They have received no information about their entitlements since their move. We decide to collect all their benefit books together and check out the position.

The Housing Manager begins by telling Eric that he should be making a record of every act of vandalism, noting the day and the time and the names of the perpetrators. She has no copy to hand of the information Eric has already sent them. Neither does she have any record of Emily qualifying for disability benefits: that, she says, is a matter for the Housing Benefits Officer. She sees no reason why they should not be able to move quite quickly if they can pay off their arrears, but adds that any choice they might have would be limited to unpopular areas with a high turnover of tenancies – in other words, estates just like the one they are trying to leave.

We arrive back home to find that Emily has had a visitor. A bailiff has left a warrant for Eric to appear in Court on 25 April or face arrest for non-payment of his fines.

We meet with the Housing Benefits Officer. It is soon established that Eric and Emily should not have been paying any rent over the past year. Instead of being in arrears they are in fact over £1000 in credit. Their council tax liability is similarly erased: they now owe nothing. The refund will be paid into their rent account and Eric must then write asking to be reimbursed by cheque. They might also be eligible for forty priority points for harassment. There's a real chance that they could be moving soon. I feel elated but not a flicker of emotion shows on Eric's face.

Eric and Emily have been married twenty-two years this month.

May 1996

Eric did not attend the Magistrates' Court but had paid an extra £15 off his fine. He will pay it all off when his cheque comes through from Housing.

The Housing Manager phones me at home. The Burgesses must let her know where they want to move as a matter of urgency. She has, she says aggressively, put in a lot of hard work for them over the last few weeks and doesn't now expect to have to keep chasing them up. I point out that it is only a week since they found out they could move. Moreover, they have still not received confirmation of their priority points, nor the benefits entitlement letter, nor any advice about the availability of vacant tenancies. She says there are two large packs in her office which Eric and Emily should look through. I say I will write to let them know, and immediately wonder why she doesn't do so.

Eric and Emily have received a statement of their rent account dated 1 May through the post. The balance is less than we had been quoted and there is nothing to show how it has been calculated. It is still over £1000 though. They have also received a liability order for non-payment of the council tax of £120.26 plus £33 costs for not appearing in court. They agree that I seek clarification on their behalf.

Eric wants to know what to put under 'special circumstances' on their re-housing form. I suggest he writes that Emily and Simon are vulnerable to victimisation on large estates and that they need to live in a small, supportive neighbourhood.

Two more windows, in the kitchen and a bedroom, were cracked yesterday, and 'TRAMPS' has been sprayed on their boarded up front window.

I phone the Area Housing Office. The Burgesses account has been credited with the amount we were first quoted less some outstanding payments. A full calculation will be coming some time in June. Another call to the council offices confirms that their council tax bill has now been reduced to £18.41. The clerk agrees to waive the court costs. Charges for 1996/7 have been cancelled and Mr and Mrs Burgess will be getting a letter confirming the same. I write to inform Eric and Emily.

The next time I see Eric he tells me about his visit to the Area Housing Office. He had gone to hand in their application for re-housing as the Housing Manager had demanded earlier. He had listed his preference for three small estates on the fringes of the city. When the Housing Manager read the form she had crossed through his list, saying it wasn't possible for them to move to any of those places, and had substituted three other estates (two of them large, one of them where they live at present). She had then got Eric to countersign the amendments.

Eric had called into the Area Housing Office last week to pick up his cheque and was told he would have to write them a letter. He had gone home, written it and taken it down to the town hall only to be told that the cheque had been sent to the Area Office and he would have to collect it from there. They said they would send his letter through the internal post.

Two weeks have now gone by since Eric handed in his letter at the town hall and still no cheque has arrived. Eric called into the Area Office a week ago and they claimed not to have received the letter. Fortunately I had given him a photocopy of the original so he left it with them.

Another two cars have been torched next to their house. The glass pane in their front door has been smashed and boarded up, two small panes in their kitchen window were broken at the weekend, and someone has had a go at their electricity meter on the wall outside.

Council workers have arrived to repair their outside drains. Emily and Eric have received a letter from Housing awarding them forty priority points for harassment. It does not mention the three points accrued since first they put their names down in 1993.

Eric has told the Court that he will pay his fines in full when he gets his cheque from the council. He has again been to the Area Office only to be told it would take a while to come through.

June 1996

Eric has finally taken his car to the scrapyard knowing that unless he did so it was only a matter of time before he got caught again. He feels much less stressed as a result. They are now using public transport, but finding it expensive.

Eric phones. He'd been to the Area Office again and asked about his cheque. The Housing Manager he'd been dealing with has left and her replacement only took up her post two days ago. She'd just been given the documents to process the cheque. She said it could take two weeks to come through. Six weeks have gone by already. Eric arranged to collect it from the town hall because of the impending postal strike. He'd also asked for a skip to be delivered so they could start clearing out the rubbish ready for moving.

The next time I see her Emily has had her hair cut and re-styled ready for her fiftieth birthday. It has cost her £23 but she looks a treat. We all agree it was worth every penny. She has also been for another check-up at the hospital. Her throat is still okay and she doesn't have to go again until December.

I can't believe it! Eric has had a letter from the Area Housing Office advising him that it will take another four to six weeks for their cheque to come through. We decide to write to the Chair of the Housing Committee and to their local councillor.

A bag of rubbish has been dumped in their garden.

I happen to be paying Eric and Emily a visit when a technical officer from the Area Housing Office calls to inspect their house for damage. He looks the place over in no more than three minutes, and then asks if he can speak to me outside. I agree only after Eric concurs.

The officer confides that he intends to report the house as being in an 'unsatisfactory' condition. When asked why, he refers to a bucket of urine he'd seen on the landing. That, I point out, has nothing to do with the state of the property, and remind him that it was once common practice to keep a chamber pot under the bed. The Burgesses bathroom is downstairs. I offer to let him have an account of the family's four years of persistent victimisation and how it has brought them down. He agrees to fill the form in 'conditionally' pending my letter.

Eric is angry and hurt when I tell them what the officer had said. They agree to me writing a similar letter to the one we sent to their local councillor. We also dig out a photograph of their living room taken a few months after they had moved in when it had been newly decorated. The print is date-stamped, and we decide to enclose it with the letter.

We then pay a visit to the Area Housing Office and are admitted almost immediately to see the new Housing Manager, a friendly and respectful woman. Because she'd only been in the job a few days she couldn't say why Eric and Emily had been waiting so long for their cheque. A letter had gone to the City Treasurer on 7 June and it should take no longer than two weeks for the cheque to be sent to them.

The Housing Manager also tells us about a bungalow that has become available on a small estate. She wonders if Eric and Emily would be interested. It sounds just what they are looking for and we arrange a viewing.

Eric smiles for the first time.

Later in the day the Housing Manager phones me full of apologies. She has learned that the bungalow is designated for older people only. She asks if I will let the Burgesses know; I tell her that it's her responsibility. She says she will try to put a card through their door later today. I post them a quick note just in case.

Over the weekend, Emily has been packing in readiness for moving; even Simon has been sorting out his bedroom. She wants to enrol for a new college course but is waiting until they are settled in a new house. The skip they ordered has still not appeared.

Last Monday they had called at social services for a disability bus pass but the office had no record of Emily being registered as disabled. They had been told to enquire at the Disability Section whose office is

eight miles away. They'd taken a bus only to find it has irregular hours
and was shut when they got there.

Oh, what next! Eric and Emily have been caught without a TV
licence by a detector van. They agree to me writing a letter explaining
their circumstances and enclosing proof of the cheque they were
expecting from the council.

Still no cheque – nearly a week after the date promised by the
Housing Manager on our last visit and two months since all this began.
We decide to call at the town hall. The cashier makes a phone call and
then informs Eric that the cheque has been stopped by the Area
Housing Office: Eric, he says, will have to contact them to find out why.
We are momentarily stunned, and then I feel a silent rage welling
inside. I begin to understand what drives people into attacks on officials.

We ring the Area Office from a call box. The Housing Manager says
she told us the cheque would be paid 'in all good faith'. She thinks it
may have been stopped by the Area Housing Manager because of the
repairs judged necessary to the house: he is out of the office at present.
The call cost 50p.

The next day I phone again with the Burgesses' permission. Apparently
the cheque has been stopped because 'repairs might be needed to the
house'. Also, I am told, Mr Burgess has failed to report all the broken
windows. I point out they've had so many broken that they now feel
safer behind boards. The Housing Manager went on to say that, of
course, they could have the money immediately if they elected not to
move.

We need to know the legal position. Eric and Emily give me permission to contact the Housing Advice Centre on their behalf. The
Housing Rights Adviser suggests we first write to the Area Housing
Manager demanding to know within seven days why the cheque has
been stopped. Failing a satisfactory reply we should then either consult
a solicitor through Legal Aid or write to the Ombudsman. I copy the
letter to the Chair of the Housing Committee.

An Environmental Health Officer contacts me to arrange a visit to
Eric and Emily's in order to assess the physical condition of the property. Emily phones me later the same day to say they have been offered
a property to view next Tuesday morning.

July 1996

Eric and Emily have been busy cleaning and tidying. They are really
excited at the prospect of a move. I arrange to meet them to view the

house at 10:00 am tomorrow, after they have collected the keys from the Housing Office. It had been Emily's birthday yesterday but she'd received no presents.

Next morning I locate the new house and wait outside as arranged. Arriving early gives me time to suss out the neighbourhood. It looks promising. The houses opposite are privately owned and decked with hanging baskets in flower. The gardens are more than neat, they're manicured. There's a greenhouse, intact, and a number of new cars parked in the small street. The house the Burgesses are viewing is the middle of five, three-storey properties with integral garages and standing space at the front. Each house has a long, narrow back garden with a fence and gate at the bottom beyond which is open ground leading to a river. The grass has been newly trimmed by the council and there is no rubbish anywhere. I see neighbours waving and talking to each another: one of them tells me the street is the quietest on the estate.

When the Burgesses have still not arrived by 11:00 am, I phone the Housing Office who confirm they had collected the keys. Soon afterwards I see Eric, Emily and Simon walking down the path: Jack's car was out of petrol so he'd been unable to give them a lift. They'd had to bus the ten miles from their house to the Housing Office and then catch another to the estate.

Eric has learned that the houses are soon to have new kitchens and double glazing. Gas central heating has recently been installed. Both sets of neighbours pop in to introduce themselves and have a chat. The family one side has lived there ten years and the other thirteen years. One of the women is the secretary of the local tenants' association and runs a social group for nine- to fourteen-year-olds.

As we drive into town I ask Simon if the house is better or worse than he'd imagined: 'better', he says. Emily too is thrilled by it, especially the size. Eric is quiet and thoughtful: a lot of internal redecoration is needed and curtains and carpets would be expensive. He'll make up his mind when Jack and Annie have seen it. They have just two days to decide. I suggest we check if they are eligible for a decoration grant and a community care grant.

The next day I arrive at Eric and Emily's house at 1:30 pm – the man from Environmental Health is due at 2:00 pm. The house is tidy and the family are smartly turned out. We go over the good and bad points of the new house. Jack is going to see it tomorrow before they have to take the keys back and give their decision.

At 2:10 pm a Mr Rideout from Environmental Health knocks on the door. He makes a careful inspection of the property, inside and out, with Eric, Emily, Simon and me all following in tow. He says the house should have been pulled down years ago. We are all aware that every window, except the one in Eric and Emily's bedroom, has been broken and boarded up. Although the state of the property hasn't improved since the Burgesses moved in, he says, neither has it got any worse. As we stand looking at the house from the back garden, a young lad walks up the path as if it was a public right of way. Mr Rideout is visibly taken aback.

It's a couple of days before I see Emily and Eric again. They have said yes to the new house and signed a tenancy agreement. Eric was asked to sign a re-housing form at the same time and, when he asked why, was told it is standard procedure. They have been given four days in which to move. Eric has asked for an extra week. The housing official has warned them that they will have to pay rent on both properties until they return the keys for their old house.

Jack is so taken with the new house that he's decided not to move into a flat of his own, as he'd planned, but to stay with his mum and dad. He's going to make his bedroom really smart.

A week goes by. They have still heard nothing about their cheque and want me to phone Housing. The Area Housing Manager tells me that he has processed an emergency cheque for £547 which should be through in two weeks time. He is holding back the remaining £500 to pay for 'enzyme treatment and maybe other small repairs'. The balance will be sent on when this work is completed. He will let me know when the cheque can be collected. I mention the skip the Burgesses ordered some time ago and he promises to see to it immediately.

I suggest to Eric and Emily that we should start thinking about Simon's schooling. With their permission, I phone the Special Needs Section of the Education Department to ask if Simon could attend a local, mainstream school with extra teaching support after they move. The official asks me to submit in writing the reasons why such an option might be better for Simon.

Emily and Eric have decided to stay in their old house another week as they are still not ready for moving. Now they have two lots of rent to pay, their cheque has not surfaced, and there's no sign of the skip. They have had a letter from the TV Licensing Authority in reply to my submission advising that they would not be summonsed provided their licence is renewed with effect from the beginning of July.

Eric asks if I would enquire about their emergency cheque at the town hall – and the skip. The cashier tells me a cheque is awaiting collection, although no-one has seen fit to notify Eric and Emily. It is now almost three months since they were first informed of the surplus in their rent account. A housing official finally confesses that the council discontinued providing skips to tenants some time ago.

A Parent Liaison Officer from the Education Department rings in response to my letter about Simon. He says he'll contact the local school to find out the position. Almost immediately someone else from the Special Needs Section phones. Her attitude is to blame the family for Simon's failure to take up the place reserved for him at special school. I point out that Simon's statement specifically recommended that work would need to be done with the family before Simon could be re-integrated into school, and that such support had not been provided. She informs me that she had ceased to maintain the statement and that Simon no longer had a place at the special school. She intended to refer him to a special unit 'for kids not attending school'. I remind her that she will have to write and explain her decision to the Burgesses.

Eric and Emily phone. They'd been to the town hall to collect their cheque. It had been made out for the full sum of £1050 – without anything being held back against the possible cost of repairs and 'enzyme treatment'. It was also dated 12 June, erasing the past five weeks of waiting and chasing at a stroke. Eric had said nothing, pocketed the cheque, and banked it on his way to phone me. We have four long days to wait to see if it clears.

A Social Fund Officer rings me about Eric and Emily's application for a community care grant and loan to help with removal costs and the replacement of damaged curtains and carpets. Although sympathetic to their plight, she is not happy about allowing money for this purpose. In the end, she agrees to authorise a community care grant towards removal costs and a nominal sum for three sets of curtains, and to offer a loan for carpets. I'm left pondering the way such claims are decided, sure in my own mind that the Burgesses would not have received anything without someone like me to speak for them.

Four days after Eric and Emily picked up their cheque from the town hall, an envelope is pushed through their letter box. Inside is a cheque for £550 – the emergency cheque promised by the Area Housing Manager! Eric calmly says he'll be taking it back, unfazed by yet another administrative cockup. They have now paid the bulk of the fines they'd incurred on their old car and purchased a new TV licence.

Annie is pregnant again. This time it's Ben's baby.

A fax comes through at work from the Area Housing Manager asking the Burgesses or me to contact him urgently or risk having the new tenancy withdrawn. By the time I phone him he has already been round to see Eric and Emily. He'd told them that they are not entitled to housing benefit in respect of the new house until they have taken up residence and handed over the keys to their old let. He is concerned that the Burgesses might incur liability for any damage caused to the empty property while they are holding two tenancies. I cannot help thinking his worries on that score have arisen some four years too late.

He also reproaches the Burgesses for having cashed the cheque they were inadvertently given knowing that the council had intended to retain £500 against any repairs that might be needed to their old house. While acknowledging that Mr Burgess has now returned the emergency cheque for £550 to the City Treasurer's, he says he intends to recommend that the council commence recovery action against them. I point out forcefully that the Burgesses had only claimed what was rightfully theirs, and that the only written information they had ever received specifically referred to their overpayment of £1050. I suggest that if the Burgesses are found to owe the council money after they have exchanged tenancies then they should be sent a detailed invoice like anyone else.

The Parent Liaison Officer phones from the Education Department to say that the Burgesses would soon be receiving a letter informing them that Simon's statement is not being maintained because he hasn't attended school. They have the right to appeal but this could take up to six months. In the meantime, when a place becomes available, he could attend the Pupil Referral Service Unit where he would work in a small group until he was ready to be helped back into mainstream education.

Eric and Emily have arranged to move on the first Saturday in August. They have to return their house keys to the local Area Housing Office (a 16-mile round trip on public transport) by 12:00 noon on the following Monday or pay another full week's rent. They have been busy preparing their new house. Eric has re-plastered some of the walls ready for painting and papering. Emily has bought some new net curtains and they are going to hang them over the weekend. They have also been looking through the small ads for new furniture. Eric confirms the cheque has now been cleared. The day before it appeared in their account they had overdrawn by £18 incurring yet more bank charges, this time of £27.

Annie is now eighteen weeks pregnant and looking to move from her present accommodation. She doesn't wish to go to the mother and baby unit this time. Ricky is giving her a lot of support as Ben has upped and off. She had met Ben through the lonely hearts column of the local newspaper.

August 1996

Children are playing in the street. Emily opens the front door of their new house before I knock. We stand in the kitchen and I am made to feel self-conscious by the brightness flooding into the house after the months of sitting with barely a chink of light showing through the boards that had previously shuttered their broken windows. They have draped every window with new net curtains and are looking to buy a blind for the kitchen. I suspect they too are feeling rather exposed.

Simon is eager to show me round and Emily tells me he's been getting up early and going to bed early since they moved. Today he's been dressed since 7:30 am.

I had been on holiday when they moved and I could see they'd been busy in the interim. Eric's first job had been to fit a dimmer switch in the living room, as if at last they feel able to exercise some control over their lives. He'd put up ceiling tiles, insulated the floor, taken a scythe to the lawn and mended the back gate. They had bought some plastic chairs and a table which would double for use in the kitchen and the garden. A new kitchen worktop had been fitted by the council. They have new curtains in the living room and Eric shows me how they tie back.

Members of Emily's family have also stepped in to help. Her mother has given them her three-piece suite, a large display cabinet, a shower unit and a new bed for Simon, and her sister has given them a dining table. Two nephews had lent a hand with the move. The Burgesses have had little contact with their wider family over the past few years. People were reluctant to visit them on their strife-torn estate in the conditions in which they were living, and their bunker-like existence had turned them in on themselves. The re-emergence of these ties augurs well for the future.

Eric and Emily show me a letter they have received from Housing saying their council tax bill now stands at £352. Crossing my fingers, I reassure them that the amount will be reduced once their benefits are credited to them at their new address. On my way out, I notice their TV licence standing in a frame on top of the TV. 'So we don't forget', says Eric.

As I drive away I see them through my rear-view mirror talking to a

neighbour over the garden fence. For the first time I feel the faint stir-
rings of hope. Things seem to be on the up.

I phone the education official named by the Parent Liaison Officer
as the person who will be contacting the Burgesses regarding the revo-
cation of Simon's statement. There's been a change of plan. As I am
involved with the Burgesses, it has been decided to maintain the statement and to give the family until Christmas to get Simon back into
school. The Pupil Referral Service will provide transport when a place
becomes available. She suggests I get in touch with them at the beginning of term to find out if there is a vacancy for Simon.

September 1996

Annie may have to go into the mother and baby unit after all as she still
has rent arrears and won't be able to get her own flat in time for the
birth of her baby.

I phone the Pupil Referral Service as advised. They have had a letter
from the principal officer in charge of Special Needs but no information about the Burgesses, not even their new address, and no copy of
Simon's statement. I briefly outline the difficulties the family has experienced, on the basis of which the adviser says she thinks Simon sounds
more like 'an anxious non-attender' than a lad with behavioural difficulties as she had been told. In that case, she says, a special school
would be an inappropriate placement for him, and she talks about
setting up an individual programme of integration, starting with short-
term tuition at home, aimed at settling him at a school in the locality.

I relay all this information to Eric and Emily and we discuss the
choice of schools, finally settling on a preferred option. They ask me if I
will make the initial contact with the headmaster. He is amiable and
helpful and suggests an early meeting with Simon and his parents.

I call to collect the three of them for the appointment with the headmaster. On the way, Emily tells me that she has been to visit Annie who
still hasn't been round to see them since they moved. Emily and Eric are
upset by her distancing herself so. Emily is hoping that she might move
near to them one day.

The school is small, pleasantly located and friendly feeling. We spend
an hour talking with the headmaster. He is surprised the Burgesses have
never been given a copy of Simon's statement and says he'll ring the
Special Needs Section to have a copy sent to them. By rights, he says,
parents should have a chance to add their own comments to the state-

ment and to approve what others have written about their child. He concludes the interview by offering Simon a place at the school.

Two days later the Pupil Referral Service confirm their plan for Simon. They will provide five and a half hours home tuition a week for two weeks; a further period of personal tuition somewhere neutral like a library; and then re-integrate Simon into school on a part-time basis in the first instance.

Emily has registered to do four courses at FE college: two before Christmas on verbal communication and time skills, and two more in the New Year on money skills and listening for pleasure. She had taken herself by bus to the college to register. It is the first time she has been anywhere without Eric for a long time.

The home tutor arrives for her first session at 10:00 am. She spends an hour and a half with Simon and when finally they emerge both look pleased with themselves. Simon had been busy on the laptop computer. As the tutor leaves she gives me a package from the Pupil Referral Service. It is Simon's statement along with a note explaining that, as no specific mention is made in it of the special school to which he was supposed to be referred, the way is clear for him to take up the place he has been offered. I read the documents out to Eric, Emily and Simon. Eric pronounces himself pleased that Simon has taken 'the first steps to learning again'.

October 1996

I can see that the priorities Eric and Emily had set themselves in the early part of the year have almost been fulfilled. They have moved to a house where they can settle and plan for the future. Simon is being helped back into mainstream school and Emily has enrolled at the nearby FE college. Eric, relieved of many of the pressures that have been bearing down on him for so long, has begun to find time for himself, setting about the house and garden, and planning how the kitchen should look after the council has fitted the new units. He has also renewed his long-standing interest in the paranormal and is doing quite a bit of reading on the subject. Family photos have been brought out in new frames and all their ornaments and books are now unpacked and on display. I sense the tensions and fears which have gripped the family for at least the last four years are slowly loosening their hold. I too have begun to feel more relaxed.

One sunny morning a call comes through to me at work from their neighbour. Eric Burgess killed himself this morning.

FACING UP TO SYSTEM ABUSE

The story of our involvement – still ongoing – with the Burgesses has been recounted at length and in detail in order to show the disabling effects that system abuse can have on families and to illustrate the important part that advocacy has to play in enabling them to resist its threat. System abuse is more a cumulative process than a one-off event: a wearing down rather than an assault. Its drip-drip effects are only properly revealed over time and only properly documented through close acquaintance with people's daily lives.

System abuse shows itself when people's problems are made worse by the services that are intended to support them. As an umbrella term, it refers to institutional attitudes, policies and practices that hurt children, harm family integrity or infringe basic rights (Gil, 1982). System abuse is not perpetrated by any single person nor is it the consequence of any single act. It is a faceless phenomenon that eludes simple attempts to pin it down in terms of who, what, where and when. System abuse is best seen as arising, often unwittingly, from the impersonal workings of the bureaucratic machine.

A huge amount of effort has been put into investigating physical and sexual abuse. By contrast, there has been very little research into what Cooper *et al.* (1987) describe as 'the plaguing problem of system abuse'. There are probably all sorts of reasons for this omission. Official agencies are more prone to secrecy than openness about their own failings, and whistle-blowers are often dealt with harshly. In any case, system abuse usually arises as a result of the actions of more than one agency. Only those affected may see the full picture and they usually lack the power to speak out or, when they do, their voices go unheard. Because system abuse has a long fuse, it is hard to link cause and effect without close knowledge of an individual or family's personal history. Without such a perspective it is all too easy to mistake the signs of system abuse for something else. For instance, problems encountered by parents with learning difficulties are frequently put down to their own limitations when they owe more to deficiencies in the support services (Booth and Booth, 1994a).

The Burgess family are a case in point. Many of the problems they encountered throughout the period covered by the research diary arose directly out of their dealings with the service system:

- All the family were trapped in a substandard house and condemned to live in what for them was the equivalent of a war zone – where they were blitzed by vandalism and stalked by fear – as the result of an administrative error on the part of the Housing Department which not only erroneously put them in arrears with their rent but also obliged them to manage on less money than was their due.

- Although Emily had been assessed as needing long-term help, her social worker and support worker were withdrawn and not replaced – when they were referred to a new area social services team after moving house – with deleterious effects on her personal motivation and the general management of the household.
- The Education Department's failure to fulfil the recommendations in Simon's statement, particularly for someone to work with the family, was crucially implicated in him missing two valuable years of schooling. The victimisation of the family also cut Simon off from boys and girls his own age, left him without friends, virtually confined him to the house or the company of his parents, and affected his health (as shown by his bed-wetting).
- No-one listened to Eric's concerns about how Annie was being sexually exploited. She ended up getting pregnant by a Schedule 1 offender while temporarily in the care of the local authority. Finally, she lost her child at least in part because her parents' own housing situation prevented them from giving her the shelter and security she and her baby needed.

System abuse is best revealed in the details of people's everyday encounters with street-level bureaucrats and the front-line representatives of authority. It is precisely through these incidents and exchanges – the experience of 'one dammed thing after another' – that people like the Burgesses come to feel the system is against them. Their generic quality is illustrated by the instances when the police asked Eric and Emily what they had been doing to provoke the vandals who had damaged their car, and later suggested they should take more care of their house and themselves so as not to attract trouble. They were made to feel as though they were at fault when the real problem rested with the landlord and the law. Blaming the victim is a typical form of system abuse.

The characteristic features of system abuse may be picked up through the experience of those for whom it is a pressing reality. Prosser (1992) has begun the task of producing such an ethnography. He interviewed parents who had been caught up in child protection proceedings and uses their accounts to identify a list of common complaints about agency practices and the behaviour of practitioners that he summarises under the heading of system abuse. This list includes: failing to involve people in decisions affecting them; adding to the problems already faced by families; seeing only evidence that confirms prior opinions; forming snap judgements on the basis of partial enquiries; failing to look at individuals in their wider family and social context; and treating people as ciphers. Among the specific examples of system abuse that Prosser cites are: practitioners who interpret their role idiosyncratically and fail to follow laid-down procedures or who adopt a dogmatic stance regarding the interpretation of evidence and refuse to listen to other points of view; the misuse of confidential information; poor agency co-operation; and experts who deviate from their field of expertise.

As Prosser's list makes clear, system abuse is a form of bad practice. But where bad practice does not always damage those it afflicts, system abuse does – either because the individual or family is particularly vulnerable or because the bad practice is particularly serious or sustained. The Burgesses file shows such a process at work and enables us to pick out aspects of their treatment at the hands of the service system that impaired their family functioning, undermined their competence, impacted adversely on the children, increased their stress and contributed to their experience of system abuse.

Unforeseen effects of intervention

Emily's efforts to keep in touch with her daughter after Annie had been temporarily admitted to a children's home resulted in her running up a phone bill that they were unable to pay, getting cut off, so losing regular contact with Annie and losing their link with the support services. When Annie eventually returned home, Eric and Emily noticed a big change in her personality. She had become aggressive and demanding and altogether more difficult to manage. They received no counselling or advice on how to deal with her behaviour.

Maladministration

The failure of officials to forward the Burgesses records to their new Area Office when they moved house resulted in them being charged excess rent for over a year, precipitated budgetary problems, debt, court cases (for non-payment of fines and council tax) and a serious risk of imprisonment, and caused enormous extra stress which ate away at family relationships and further eroded their capacity to cope.

Passing the buck

Constantly being referred backwards and forwards between officials, offices, and departments convinces people that they are up against the system. Eric was bounced between his Area Housing Office and the town hall many times – each trip involving a lengthy and costly bus ride across the city – as he strove to get his hands on the cheque he was owed. Social services staff sent Emily on an 8-mile bus ride in pursuit of her disability pass only for her to find the office was shut when she arrived. The police refused to do anything about the constant harassment on the grounds that the Burgesses would not sign a statement naming the culprits.

Unrealistic demands

The Housing Department was slow to respond to the Burgesses pressing need to escape the victimisation that was blighting their lives yet when finally a property was offered they were required to make a decision within 24 hours and to move within four days of accepting the tenancy. When they failed to complete the move in the time allowed they were billed on both properties.

Double standards

One of the reasons given for removing Annie temporarily into care was school non-attendance. Eric had been keeping her at home for her own safety because of his fears that she had fallen into the clutches of a paedophile ring. However, after admitting her to a children's home, the local authority was able to provide her with schooling for only two days a week. In a similar vein, whereas the local authority took three months to repay without interest money owed to the Burgesses, they in turn incurred heavy bank charges for going into the red for one day while waiting for the local authority cheque to clear.

Lack of involvement in decisions

The failure to involve people in decisions affecting their lives leads them into thinking things are going on behind their back and feeling as if they are up against the system. When Annie was taken temporarily into care, Eric and Emily did not receive any written minutes of the outcomes of her first three reviews. As parents and grandparents, they were not involved at all in any of the proceedings leading up to Billy's adoption, although Annie was still a minor. Equally, Eric and Emily were never sent a copy of Simon's statement of educational needs although legally they should have been given a chance to add their own comments.

Poor communication

The Burgesses were hampered in coping with their troubles by the regular flow of duff information given them by officials. The episode of the skip is symptomatic of this problem. Three times they ordered a skip from the council so they could clear the rubbish from their house (including the store of missiles hurled through their windows which they had kept as evidence) prior to moving. Three times they followed up their request and were assured a skip was on its way: on the last occasion the Area Housing Manager promised to 'see to it' himself. After a month of hanging on they were told the council had stopped providing skips for tenants.

Information was hard to obtain at the best of times without knowing exactly what and whom to ask. Even so, the information given was often contradictory (as when the Special Needs Co-ordinator told Eric and Emily that transport would be provided for Simon to attend the Pupil Referral Unit only to be countermanded later by the Pupil Referral Service); insufficient (as when they were not told the cheque due them had been stopped, or provided with a statement of how the sum owed them had been calculated); or inaccurate (as when arrangements were made for them to view a bungalow which it later transpired was only available for letting to elderly people or when they were wrongly sent a final demand for council tax of £352 instead of the £18 they were actually liable). Letters frequently went unanswered. The six letters we wrote together to the Chair of the Housing Committee and to their ward councillor about their housing and rent problems elicited not a single written reply. Poor communication adds to the sense of the system as a citadel that needs to be scaled. People such as the Burgesses lack the resources with which to mount a sustained and effective attack.

Inaccessibility of practitioners

Eric and Emily found it very hard to get in touch with practitioners when they felt in need of help or advice. Having to use public phones made the task doubly difficult and very expensive. Often they would ring only to find the worker was out of the office or, more frustratingly, in the building but away from their desk. Where people had their own extensions their office colleagues usually did not answer them. Switchboard operators did not take messages. In any case, no-one could return their calls. On countless occasions they were told the person they were seeking would be back in the office 'at 2:00 pm' or could be contacted 'first thing in the morning' only to find, after trooping to the phone box again, that he had 'changed his schedule' or that she was 'out on an emergency' or 'caught up in a meeting'.

Lack of continuity in service delivery

Support when provided was always insecure and liable to cease without regard to the continuing needs of the family. Staff turnover was one cause of such discontinuities. The Burgesses had to deal with three different Area Housing Managers in the course of one year. Such comings and goings frequently contribute to a failure of 'institutional memory' (Bunker, 1978) as experienced workers leave, taking with them their detailed case knowledge. They also lead to idiosyncratic changes or contradictions in the interpretation of policy. One Housing Manager insisted the Burgesses could only move into another hard-to-let property, while her successor imposed no such limitation.

Poor co-ordination also makes for muddles and mistakes. When the Burgesses moved into a new housing district, their records were not transferred from their previous office with the result that their housing benefit was stopped. This move also brought them under a new social work team which did not replace their social worker or their support worker After a lengthy delay, without ever receiving a visit, they were simply notified that their file had been closed. This illustrates the point that system abuse often occurs despite the best efforts of individual practitioners. Eric and Emily received valuable and valued support from their social worker and support worker whom they liked and who in turn demonstrated a genuine commitment to helping the family. During their time with the Burgesses these workers had sorted out their benefits, secured them grants for decorating and household equipment, arranged day trips and holidays for them, fixed Emily up at college, and generally given the family a sense of purpose. The damage to the family resulting from the loss of this support came about because of blips in the working of the system rather than culpability on the part of any one individual.

Other reasons for the falling away of support are less easy to explain.

The educational welfare officer assigned to tackle Simon's non-attendance at school by walking him there in a morning stopped calling when he would not get up. No attempt was made to address this problem with the family and no follow-up action was taken. Simon was just left to lie in bed.

Blaming the parents for deficits in the services

Simon's refusal to go to school and his parent's reluctance to make him were tied up with his fear of being bullied and the family's experience of victimisation. Yet no-one who was in a position to help – from Education, Housing, Social Services or the police – was prepared to acknowledge this fact or face up to its consequences. Instead, the problem was thrown back at Eric and Emily and couched in terms of their dysfunctional home environment and their inadequacies as parents, just as earlier they had been blamed for keeping Annie off school when no-one would take Eric's concerns about her welfare seriously. In just the same way, the Burgesses were held responsible for the state of their house (to the point of being told that they would be surcharged for any remedial work or treatment judged necessary after they had moved) despite the damage wrought by vandals and the effects of such persecution on their self-respect.

System abuse becomes more of a problem the more people lack the means to resist its pull. The fewer resources and supports people possess the more vulnerable they are to system abuse. The more they rely on the service system for support the more they risk being let down. Many people possess the adaptive capacity to absorb or shrug off the kinds of institutional failings listed above. Others have a much thinner protective layer. For people and families operating on the edge of competence, whose coping abilities are stretched, the extra burden imposed by unresponsive services may be enough to push them past breaking-point. The Burgesses belonged to this group. On their uppers, alone and isolated, their self-esteem in tatters and their motivation shot, they were unable to surmount the additional obstacles the services put in the way of their coping. They needed an advocate.

ADVOCACY IN ACTION

Advocacy is about working with people to support them in ways that are responsive to their own views of their needs. When Eric and Emily agreed to join our advocacy support network they set themselves two goals: to move off the estate where they were living and to get Simon back into school. Everything that followed between us was defined by their purpose and geared to these ends.

The Burgesses story, as presented in the research diary of our relationship, illustrates many of the ways in which an advocate can help a family to combat the threat of system abuse. At one time or another, sometimes simultaneously, the following roles have come to the fore:

- *Advocate as witness* – simply being there is often enough. 'Being there' is not about acting for parents but about lending them authority. Even this passive support empowers people and makes them feel that they can get things done. Knowing there is someone there watching what they are doing also helps to keep officials and practitioners on their toes and deters them from taking advantage of people who are seen as too weak to fight back.
- *Advocate as buffer* – helping to absorb some of the pressures on the family by fielding or deflecting matters that might exacerbate their troubles or stress.
- *Advocate as voice* – making sure the parents' side of the story is represented and their views are heard.
- *Advocate as go-between* – helping to facilitate and improve liaison between the family, practitioners and the services.
- *Advocate as interpreter* – translating officialese into language the parents can understand and otherwise making information accessible to them.
- *Advocate as listener* – reducing parents' feelings of isolation by enabling them to share their worries, air their grievances or just talk things over.
- *Advocate as scribe* – writing letters and helping with form-filling.
- *Advocate as problem-solver* – helping parents to identify the choices they face in dealing with their problems and then supporting them in their decisions, and also ensuring that practitioners are apprised of options they may have missed.
- *Advocate as fixer* – sorting out problems of service delivery caused by poor co-ordination, errors, oversights and the like.
- *Advocate as conduit* – channelling the lessons learned in supporting one family for the benefit of another.
- *Advocate as sounding-board* – encouraging families to have confidence in their own ability to cope by helping them to work things out for themselves.

- *Advocate as confidante* – someone with whom private and confidential information can be safely shared in the sure knowledge that it will not be passed on or used against the family.
- *Advocate as ally* – someone who is unambiguously on the family's side, prepared to stand by them, and whose actions are always consistent with this stance.

The Burgesses' story also highlights some of the constraints on the role of the advocate. An advocate cannot change local authority policies or practices that impact unfairly on families; make professionals like them or treat them with respect; undo the harm done by deficiencies in the services and support provided to families; shield people from discrimination and day-to-day harassment; or change the attitudes that fuel their victimisation in the community. Equally, an advocate cannot erase past hurts or ensure a future free from distress. For families like the Burgesses, life will ever be a succession of problems. Experience tells them there are always more around the corner. An advocate can try to relieve some of the external pressures – such as system abuse – that bear down on them, but cannot give them inner peace. Eric Burgess' untimely death is a sad reminder of the limits of advocacy.

Chapter 10

Where next?

Drawing out the lessons our research holds for policy and practice presents us with something of a dilemma. Do we emphasise the differences or the similarities between our study families and others? Highlighting the parents' learning difficulties risks diverting attention from the fact that many of the problems and disadvantages their children had experienced came about for other reasons. We said at the beginning that our study promised to throw new light on the process of parenting itself, not just on a particular group of parents. The same is true of the lessons which emerge, some of which properly apply to all families and children in need.

RISK AND RESILIENCE

More effort has gone into studying the damage children suffer as a result of poor parenting than has been put into studying those who overcome the disadvantages of their upbringing. Yet this study has shown that not all children are victims of their situation and many demonstrate considerable adaptability in coping with lives filled with difficulty. As the experience of the now-adult people in the study clearly demonstrates, children's destinies are not fixed by having a mother or father with learning difficulties. From this perspective, the focus of interest shifts away from the nature of the risks they face to the source of their resilience.

Paying more attention to the sources of resilience in children is important because it promises to open up new ways in which they might be helped to overcome the hazards of their upbringing. The risk paradigm encourages practitioners to look for what is going wrong rather than what is going right in the lives of children. It is not surprising that people trained to look for problems usually manage to find them. This is why the at-risk label, like other negative labels, might itself be regarded as a risk factor. We need to know what it is that makes children prevail as well as what makes them succumb under conditions of risk. We shall be better placed to develop forms of preventive support, and ways of promoting positive outcomes for children and young people, if we learn more about *why* some children are not damaged by a deprived childhood and *what* factors help them to rise above their disadvantages.

The notion of resilience as a compensatory factor shielding children from the potentially harmful effects of parenting deficits calls for a reappraisal of the meaning of parental competence itself.

PARENTAL COMPETENCE

Parental competence is widely equated with parentcraft. From this standpoint, good-enough parents are endowed with the skills required to meet their child's developmental needs while inadequate parents lack these skills. By this reasoning, (in)competence is located as a characteristic of the parent which can be assessed in terms of the child's developmental progress.

This study has shown that no such simple link between parenting skills and child outcomes can be assumed. How children turn out depends on more than just their parents. Parents are not the only people involved in bringing up children. Lots of others play a part – from brothers and sisters, grandparents, aunts, uncles and other relatives, through to nannies, childminders, neighbours, friends and peers, teachers and still more distant influences. It is clear from the life stories of the now-adult children in this study that the strength of their parents' support system had an important bearing on their experience of growing up.

Competence may more properly be seen as a distributed feature of parents' social network rather than as an individual attribute. The notion of what might be termed 'distributed competence' attests to the fact that parenting is mostly a shared activity and acknowledges the interdependencies that comprise the parenting task. From this point of view, parental competence is actually resourced by the family's social network. It is also vulnerable to changes over time in the relationships that make up this network. The birth of another child, the death of a grandparent, a change of school, the separation of parents, the onset of unemployment, a move to a new house can all affect the capacity of the family and social network to sustain or support parents in their parenting. Parental competence, then, is not a fixed ability but is crucially related to the way people live and can only be understood or assessed in the context of their lives. Just as resilience is better understood as a feature of the life course than an attribute of the person so competence too is better viewed as a process than a skill.

To date, the skills-model of competence has led to most effort going into developing methods and programmes of parenting training. Most of these have been based on a social learning model or behavioural principles (Smith and Pugh, 1996). Their aim has been to train parents, more often mothers, in the skills they lack. The notion of 'distributed competence' – competence as a distributed feature of a family's social network – directs our attention to the fact that child outcomes are not just a function of the skills or lack of skills of parents. On the one hand, you have the situation where the family's social network compensates for the parents' lack of skills – as typified by the supportive grandmother. On the other hand, you have the situation where a parent's skills are undermined by the weakness of their social network – as, for example, in the case of a single mother with no family or friends to call on, struggling to make ends meet in bad housing, and pestered by predatory men. The notion of 'distributed competence' obliges us to look at parenting in context rather than at mothers and fathers as individuals. It requires us to attend to the family as a unit rather than to individual members. It suggests that parents and children are best supported in the context of their own extended families, neighbourhoods and communities. And it obliges us to address the environmental pressures in their lives that make their coping more difficult. These tasks call for forms of support other than just training – forms of support that draw on the lessons of the advocacy movement and of community development.

THE IMPORTANCE OF FAMILY

The study underscores three crucial aspects of the role of the family in helping children overcome the disadvantages of their childhood and establish a berth in the adult world.

First, family ties can nurture resilience in children. A key protective factor shielding children from a disadvantaged upbringing is a positive attachment to at least one adult apart from their parents who shows them unconditional acceptance (McIntyre et al., 1990; Werner, 1993). Such supportive relationships are most often found within the extended family.

Second, family supports may compensate for a lack of competence on the part of the parents in order to ensure satisfactory care for the child. A significant predictor of child well-being is the adequacy of supports that parents have regardless of their own parenting skills (Tymchuk, 1992). A key source of such supports is the extended family. These ties need to be reinforced, not undermined or displaced, by professional intervention.

Third, adults need parents too. For most of the now-adult children with learning difficulties in the study, their relationship with their mother and/or father provided the only close, secure and continuing emotional bond in their lives. Even for those without learning difficulties, this relationship lay at the heart of their adult identity. This point has a bearing on the interpretation of the 'paramountcy principle' enshrined in the Children Act 1989. This principle binds the courts into giving paramount consideration to the welfare of the child when determining any matter relating to his or her upbringing. For children born into families who need a lot of support it is tempting to invent a future in which they would be better off away from their parents. Looking back from their position in the adult world it is equally possible to see the harm that can be done by jumping too readily to any such conclusion. The question of what is in the best interests of the child always invites a response in the future tense. The true answer often appears very different in hindsight. Unable to escape these uncertainties, it is important that policy-makers and practitioners bear in mind that the state can more easily provide the supports a family needs in order to cope than it can replace the love of a child for a parent or a parent for a child. As one person in our study said, what mattered most as a child was 'the fact that we were living with people we loved'.

SOCIAL EXCLUSION

Most of the people in the study had been set apart and set upon throughout their childhood. The experience of exclusion was a common thread running through their stories. Few of those with learning difficulties had found respite in adulthood. The processes of exclusion operated on many levels.

On a personal level, people met with persistent name-calling and verbal abuse, bullying at school, and harassment and victimisation at home and in the neighbourhood. On an institutional level, the children were channelled into special schools and segregated from their peers, their parents were not listened to by people in authority, and the families were frequently subjected to forms of discriminatory treatment at the hands of official agencies sufficiently serious to warrant the label of system abuse. Economically, they were excluded by debt, unemployment, penury and the poverty trap. All these things worked together to place even greater strains on families who at the best of times had fewer personal resources on which to draw.

Social exclusion was behind many of the troubles that blotted people's childhood and beset their families. All too often these troubles are put down to the limitations of the parents when they are more properly seen as a product of their situation. The disability movement has drawn attention to the part played by social, environmental and cultural barriers in the making of disability, and has shown that the disadvantages experienced by disabled people cannot simply be explained in terms of their impairment. The effects of social exclusion on parental competence as revealed through the now-adult children in this study demonstrate how the social model of disability has equal relevance to the experience of people with learning difficulties. Recognising the impact of social exclusion is an important step forward. When problems are seen as rooted in people's personal deficits and limitations they may seem intractable and out of reach. Shifting the focus onto features of people's lives that can and should be changed challenges the negative stereotypes that inform such thinking and opens up possibilities for social action in support of families.

SUPPORTED PARENTING

The issues marked out above apply equally to all families and children in need. They point to the need for a reappraisal of much current thinking about the relationship between parental competence and child welfare. Methods of assessment based on a risk paradigm that fails to acknowledge the sources of resilience in children's lives will lower the threshold for intervention and draw an excess of families into the child protection net. A model of parental competence based on too narrow a view of the process of parenting will tend to underestimate a family's ability to cope. Practitioners who undervalue the importance of family ties are too easily led into misjudging what is in the best interests of a child. Supports must aim to tackle the damaging effects of social exclusion on family life. Such a reappraisal of policy and practice must be grounded in the lives of families in need and not in the fears of professionals.

While recognising that many of the problems encountered by

families headed by a parent or parents with learning difficulties are common among other families in need, and cannot be explained simply in terms of the parent's intellectual impairment, it is also important to acknowledge the special needs of such families. The stories we have recounted in this book (see also Booth and Booth, 1994a) bear out the lack of support provided for them. Yet the best predictor of child neglect by parents with learning difficulties 'appears to be the absence of suitable societal or familial supports' (Tymchuk, 1992). Parents will continue to fail and children will continue to suffer until we develop new forms of support that address the shortcomings in existing practices and services.

Pioneering initiatives in supported parenting in the United States (Ullmer *et al.*, 1991) have begun to piece together the elements of a new approach. The driving force behind these initiatives has been the recognition that many of the challenges encountered by professionals in supporting families stem less from the parents themselves than from deficiencies in the services (Kidd Webster, 1988). The State of Wisconsin has been among the frontrunners in this field. For over ten years, the Wisconsin Council on Developmental Disabilities (WCDD) has co-ordinated a Supported Parenting Project with the aim of helping state and local human service and public health agencies to improve the quality and effectiveness of services to families headed by parents with learning difficulties. These initiatives and programmes bear witness to a concerted attempt to address the needs of these parents and serve to highlight the lack of effort that has been put into supporting families in this country. With notable exceptions such as the Special Parenting Service in Truro (Campion, 1993; McGaw, 1993a, 1993b) and the Exeter Parenting Service (Young *et al.*, 1997) the special needs of parents with learning difficulties have been largely ignored. Over the past ten years, a great deal of systematic knowledge and practice wisdom has been gathered in Wisconsin from which much can be learned in the UK.

The idea of supported parenting is grounded on a core of practice principles that have emerged from the experience of working with mothers and fathers who have learning difficulties and their children. Foremost among these core principles are the following:

- Support must be based on respect for the parents and for the emotional bond between the parents and their children. Parents should be regarded as a resource, not as a problem.
- Parents have needs as people too.

- Support should be directed to the family as a unit rather than to individual members.
- Parents should be enabled to feel in control and to experience being competent.
- Intervention should focus on building a family's strengths rather than on attending to its weaknesses.
- Families are best supported in the context of their own extended families, neighbourhoods and communities.
- Parents must be engaged as active partners in service planning and involved as equals in choices and decisions affecting their family.

Developing programmes of support consistent with these principles has meant breaking away from the old 'deficit model' of service delivery which is resource-led and crisis-driven, focuses primarily on people's problems and failings, and puts the professional in control. By contrast, the supported parenting model involves working long term to build on a family's strengths in order to promote competence and sustain independence. The key characteristics of a more responsive and enabling support system are now better understood.

LONG-TERM SUPPORT

Parents with learning difficulties are likely to need support on a long-term, continuing basis throughout the parenting years. For workers, short-term, crisis-driven services often result in frustration, burn-out and a tendency to blame the parents. Equally, they often give rise to mistrust, despair and cyclical crisis episodes in families (Mandeville, 1992). Long-term supports foster greater mutual trust and respect, improve the ways that families use support, allow more opportunities for preventive work, and enable a more holistic approach (Hoffman *et al.*, 1990).

TRUSTING RELATIONSHIPS

A positive relationship between parent and practitioner is a crucial ingredient of effective support and a primary goal of intervention. Many parents will have had bad experiences of the services in the past. Overcoming their suspicions may be a lengthy process. Breaking down these barriers calls for a genuine appreciation of the parents as people and a readiness to get involved with the family. Parents 'know when you don't like them and they know when you don't like their children'

(Snodgrass, 1992). The values and attitudes that practitioners hold exert a more important influence on family outcomes than their knowledge and skills (Espe-Sherwindt and Kerlin, 1990).

MAINTAINING INVOLVEMENT

The success of a support programme may depend as much on its workers' ability to involve the parents as on the abilities of the parents themselves (Espe-Sherwindt and Crable, 1993). Keeping families interested and committed is a common problem (New York State Commission on Quality of Care for the Mentally Disabled, 1993a), and one shared with most early intervention programmes (Bronfenbrenner, 1974). Life experiences that have eroded parents' sense of competence and worth are a block to participation. Also, many parents are so over-burdened by day-to-day crises that they lack the energy and personal resources to assume any more responsibilities. Two steps that have been shown by the Wisconsin Supported Parenting Project to ease these difficulties are working with parents as partners in ways that raise their self-esteem and providing practical help aimed at lightening the load on the family.

FAMILY-CENTRED SUPPORT

The children are usually the primary focus of attention for practitioners in families headed by parents with learning difficulties. The parents' own needs are often overlooked or regarded as a secondary concern. Practitioners must be prepared to adapt their priorities. Parents may be unable to meet the needs of their children unless their own needs are first addressed (Espe-Sherwindt, 1991). These needs may stem from an upbringing in which: 'No one cuddled. No one nurtured. No one cherished. No one valued. No one praised. No one played. No one supported. No one encouraged. No one comforted. No one cared. No one loved (Snodgrass, 1992)'. Or equally they may come from the effects of daily hardships visited by poverty, bad housing, exploitation, victimisation, stigma, powerlessness, isolation and the like. When support is organised from a family-centred perspective – from the point of view of what can be done to support the family rather than how to protect the child – it is more likely to be mutually agreed and less likely to be seen as threatening (Hoffman *et al.*, 1990).

INTENSIVE, IN-HOME SUPPORT

Support has been shown to be most effective where it provides the opportunity for one-to-one contact in the home. Characteristically this includes: frequent home visits, a high degree of availability, flexible scheduling, and a willingness to provide 'hands-on' help with some tasks in order to allow the parents to concentrate on more pressing ones (Hoffman *et al.*, 1990).

FLEXIBLE, INDIVIDUALISED SUPPORT

Support should be targeted on the specific needs of the family and its members. The flexibility to adjust the support to accommodate the parents' views of what help they would like is important. Similarly, where training is offered, it must be matched to the learning character-istics of the parents (Heighway, 1992). For example, parents with learning difficulties do not seem to benefit from attending groups with other parents. Adults learn from other adults 'when there is respect and trust, when they can choose what they want to learn, are motivated, and are offered support in a way and at a pace that is right for them' (Sweet, 1990).

The supported parenting model offers a way of shifting from a punitive to a positive approach to families headed by parents with learning diffi-culties. Making this shift demands a new way of thinking based on the rejection of the traditional deficit model of service delivery. In particu-lar, it calls for a switch of focus in professional practice: from people as individuals to the family as a unit; from a concentration on the assess-ment of risk and vulnerability to an even-handed appreciation of people's strengths and their resilience under pressure; from a concern about promoting dependence to the goal of building competence; from the role of expert to the role of partner. Until these changes take place, parents with learning difficulties will continue to receive rough justice and their children will continue to get a raw deal.

Bibliography

Abrams, K. (1991) 'Hearing the call of stories', *California Law Review*, 79(4), 971–1052.

Accardo, P. and Whitman, B. (1990) 'Children of mentally retarded parents', *American Journal of Diseases of Children*, 144, 69–70.

Aldridge, J. and Becker, S. (1993) *Children Who Care: Inside the World of Young Carers*, Department of Social Sciences, Loughborough: Loughborough University.

—— (1994) *My Child My Carer*, Department of Social Sciences, Loughborough: Loughborough University.

Angrosino, M. (1998) 'Mental disability in the United States: an interactionist perspective', in R. Jenkins (ed.), *Questions of Competence: Culture, Classification and Intellectual Disability*, Cambridge: Cambridge University Press.

Ariès, P. (1979) *Centuries of Childhood*, Harmondsworth: Penguin.

Ashe, M. (1989) 'Zig-zag stitching and the seamless web: thoughts on "reproduction" and the law', *Nova Law Review*, 13, 355–83.

Ashton, R. (1994) 'Introduction', in George Eliot, *Middlemarch*, Harmondsworth: Penguin.

Atkinson, D. (1988) 'Research interviews with people with mental handicaps', *Mental Handicap Research*, 1, 75–90.

Baron, J. (1991) 'The many promises of storytelling in law', *Rutgers Law Journal*, 23, 79–90.

BBC (1994) *Lost Childhoods: Children who Care for Ailing Parents*, Wednesday 4 December, BBC Radio 4.

Begun, A. (1993) 'Human behaviour and the social environment: the vulnerability, risk, and resilience model', *Journal of Social Work Education*, 29(1), 26–35.

Berrington, A. and Murphy, M. (1994) 'Changes in the living arrangements of young adults in Britain during the 1980s', *European Sociological Review*, 10, 235–57.

Bertaux, D. (1981) 'Introduction', in D. Bertaux (ed.), *Biography and Society: The Life History Approach in the Social Sciences*, London: Sage Publications.

Bertaux-Wiame, I. (1981) 'The life-history approach to the study of internal migration', in D. Bertaux (ed.), *Biography and Society: The Life History Approach in the Social Sciences*, London: Sage Publications.

Biklen, S. and Moseley, C. (1988) ' "Are you retarded?" "No, I'm Catholic": qualitative methods in the study of people with severe handicap', *Journal of the Association of Severe Handicaps*, 13, 155–62.

Birren, J. and Deutchman, D. (1991) *Guiding Autobiography Groups for Older Adults*, London: The Johns Hopkins University Press.

Bogdan, R. (1974) *Being Different: The Autobiography of Jane Fry*, New York: Wiley.

Bogdan, R. and Taylor, S. (1976) 'The judged, not the judges: an insider's view of mental retardation', *American Psychologist*, 31(1), 47–52.

Bond, H. (1995) 'When home care charges give cause for complaint', *Community Care*, 14–20 September, 23.

Booth, T. (1995) 'Sounds of still voices: issues in the use of narrative methods with people who have learning difficulties', in L. Barton (ed.), *Sociology and Disability*, London: Longmans.

Booth, T. and Booth, W. (1994a) *Parenting Under Pressure: Mothers and Fathers with Learning Difficulties*, Buckingham: Open University Press.

—— (1994b) 'For better, for worse: the prospects for partnership between professionals and parents who have learning difficulties', in T. Philpot and L. Ward (eds), *Values and Visions: Changing Ideas in Services for People with Learning Difficulties*, London: Butterworth-Heinemann.

—— (1994c) 'Parental adequacy, parenting failure and parents with learning difficulties', *Health and Social Care in the Community*, 2, 161–72.

—— (1995) 'Unto us a child is born: the trials and rewards of parenthood for people with learning difficulties', *Australia and New Zealand Journal of Developmental Disabilities*, 20(1), 25–39.

—— (1996a) 'Parental competence and parents with learning difficulties', *Child and Family Social Work*, 1(2), 81–6.

—— (1996b) 'Parenting in context: policy, practice and the Pollocks', *Child and Family Social Work*, 1(2), 93–6.

Booth, W. and Booth, T. (1993) 'Learning the hard way: practice issues in supporting parents with learning difficulties', *Social Work and Social Sciences Review*, 4(2), 148–62.

Bowen, C. (1968) *Biography: The Craft and the Calling*, Boston: Little, Brown.

Brisenden, S. (1989) 'A charter for personal care', *Progress*, 16.

Bronfenbrenner, U. (1974) 'Children, families and social policy: an American perspective', *The Family in Society: Dimensions of Parenthood*, London: HMSO.

Brooks, R. (1994) 'Children at risk: fostering resilience and hope', *American Journal of Orthopsychiatry*, 64(4), 545–53.

Bruner, J. (1987) 'Life as narrative', *Social Research*, 54(1), 11–32.

— (1990) *Acts of Meaning*, London: Harvard University Press.

—— (1991) 'The narrative construction of reality', *Critical Inquiry*, 18(1), 1–21.

Buck, F. and Hohmann, G. (1983) 'Parental disability and children's adjustment', in E. Pan, T. Backer and C. Vash (eds), *Annual Review of Rehabilitation*, Vol. 3, New York: Springer Publishing Company.

Bunker, D. (1978) 'Organizing to link social science with public policy-making', *Public Administration Review*, May–June, 223–32.

Campion, M. (1993) *Learning to be Mum*, VHS video, London: Arrowhead Productions.

Ciotti, P. (1989) 'Growing up different', *Los Angeles Times*, Part V, May 9, pp. 1, 4, 10.

Clandinin, D. and Connelly, F. (1994) 'Personal experience methods', in N. Denzin and Y. Lincoln (eds), *Handbook of Qualitative Research*, Thousand Oaks, CA: Sage.

Clough, P. (1996) ' "Again Fathers and Sons": the mutual construction of self, story and special educational needs', *Disability and Society*, 11(1), 71–81.

Cohler, B. (1987) 'Adversity, resilience and the study of lives', in E. Anthony and B. Cohler (eds), *The Invulnerable Child*, New York: The Guilford Press, pp. 363–424.

Connelly, F. and Clandinin, D. (1990) 'Stories of experience and narrative inquiry', *Educational Researcher*, 19(5), 2–14.

Cooke, A. (1980) *The Americans: Letters from America 1969–1979*, Harmondsworth: Penguin Books.

Cooper, C., Peterson, N. and Meier, J. (1987) 'Variables associated with disrupted placement in a select sample of abused and neglected children', *Child Abuse and Neglect*, 11, 75–86.

Cross, G. and Marks, B. (1995) *Parents with Learning Disabilities*, Broadstairs, Kent: Canterbury and Thanet Community Healthcare.

Denzin, N. (1989) *Interpretive Biography*, London: Sage.

Department of Health (1989) *Individuals, Programmes and Plans: Inspection of Day Services for People with a Mental Handicap*, London: Social Services Inspectorate.

Dickerson, V. and Zimmerman, J. (1993) 'A narrative approach to families with adolescents', in S. Friedman (ed.), *The New Language of Change: Constructive Collaboration in Psychotherapy*, New York: Guilford Press, pp. 226–50.

Dowdney, L. and Skuse, D. (1993) 'Parenting provided by adults with mental retardation', *Journal of Child Psychology and Psychiatry*, 34(1), 25–47.

Edgerton, R. and Bercovici, S. (1976) 'The cloak of competence: years later', *American Journal of Mental Deficiency*, 80, 345–51.

Eliot, G. (1963) 'The natural history of German life', in T. Pinney (ed.), *Essays of George Eliot*, London: Routledge and Kegan Paul.

Erikson, K. (1973) 'Sociology and the historical perspective', in M. Drake (ed.), *Applied Historical Studies*, London: Methuen, in association with Open University Press.

Espe-Sherwindt, M. (1991) 'The ISFP and parents with special needs/mental retardation', *Topics in Early Childhood Special Education*, 11(3), 107–20.

Espe-Sherwindt, M. and Crable, S. (1993) 'Parents with mental retardation: moving beyond the myths', *Topics in Early Childhood Special Education*, 13(2), 154–74.

Espe-Sherwindt, M. and Kerlin, S. (1990) 'Early intervention with parents with mental retardation: do we empower or impair?', *Infants and Young Children*, 2, 21–8.

Faraday, A. and Plummer, K. (1979) 'Doing life histories', *Sociological Review*, 27, November, 773–98.

Farmer, E. and Owen, M. (1993) *Decision-making, Intervention and Outcome in Child Protection Work*, Report to Department of Health, Bristol: University of Bristol.

Farmer, R., Rohde, J. and Sacks, B. (1993) *Changing Services for People with Learning Disabilities*, London: Chapman and Hall.

Ferrarotti, F. (1981) 'On the autonomy of the biographical method', in D. Bertaux (ed.), *Biography and Society*, London: Sage Publications.

Fisher, L. (1986) *Linked Lives: Adult Daughters and their Mothers*, New York: Harper and Row.

Flynn, M. (1986) 'Adults who are mentally handicapped as consumers: issues and guidelines for interviewing', *Journal of Mental Deficiency Research*, 30, 369–77.

Flynn, M. and Hirst, M. (1992) *This Year, Next Year, Sometime. . . . ? Learning Disability and Adulthood*, London: National Development Team and Social Policy Research Unit.

Fotheringham, J. (1980) *Mentally Retarded Persons as Parents*, unpublished manuscript, Kingston, Ontario: Department of Psychiatry, Queen's University.

Garfield, S. (1995) 'A study in life expectancy', *The Independent on Sunday*, 12 March, p. 21.

Garmezy, N. (1991) 'Resiliency and vulnerability to adverse developmental outcomes associated with poverty', *American Behavioral Scientist*, 34(4), 416–30.

Gath, A. (1988) 'Mentally handicapped people as parents', *Journal of Child Psychology and Psychiatry*, 29(6), 739–44.

Geertz, C. (1988) *Works and Lives: The Anthropologist as Author*, Stanford, CA: Stanford University Press.

Gil, E. (1982) 'Institutional abuse of children in out-of-home care', *Child and Youth Services*, 41(1–2), 7–13.

Harrington, C. and Whiting, J. (1972) 'Socialization process and personality', in Hsu, F. (ed.) *Psychological Anthropology*, Cambridge, MA: Schenkman.

Heighway, S. (1992) *Helping Parents Parent: A Practice Guide for Supporting Families Headed by Parents with Cognitive Limitations. Supported Parenting Project*, Madison: Wisconsin Council of Developmental Disabilities.

Hendrick, H. (1990) 'Constructions and reconstructions of British childhood: an interpretive survey 1800 to the present', in A. James and A. Prout (eds), *Constructing and Reconstructing Childhood: Contemporary Issues in the Sociological Study of Childhood*, London: Farmer Press.

Hirst, M. (1987) 'Careers of young people with disabilities aged between 15 and 21 years', *Disability, Handicap and Society*, 2, 61–74.

Hirst, M. and Baldwin, S. (1994) *Unequal Opportunities: Growing Up Disabled*, London: HMSO.

Hoffman, C., Mandeville, H., Kidd Webster, S., Heighway, S., Ullmer, D., Mincberg, B., Snodgrass, P., Murphy-Simon, K. and Wenger, B. (1990) *The Amelioration of Health Problems of Children with Parents with Mental Retardation 1987–1990*, Madison: Wisconsin Council on Developmental Disabilities and the Waisman Center on Mental Retardation and Human Development.

Hutson, S. and Jenkins, R. (1989) *Taking the Strain: Families, Unemployment and the Transition to Adulthood*, Buckingham: Open University Press.

James, A. and Prout, A. (eds) (1990) *Constructing and Reconstructing Childhood: Contemporary Issues in the Sociological Study of Childhood*, London: Farmer Press.

Jenkins, R. (1989) 'Barriers to adulthood: long-term unemployment and mental handicap compared', in A. Brechin and J. Walmsley (eds), *Making Connections: Reflecting on the Lives and Experiences of People with Learning Difficulties*, London: Hodder and Stoughton.

Jenks, C. (ed.) (1982) *The Sociology of Childhood*, London: Batsford.

Johnson, P. and Clark, S. R. (1984) 'Service needs of developmentally disabled parents', in J. Berg and J. de Jong (eds), *Perspectives and Progress in Mental Retardation*, Vol. 1, Baltimore: University Park Press.

Jones, G. (1995) *Leaving Home*, Buckingham: Open University Press.

Jones, G. and Wallace, C. (1992) *Youth, Family and Citizenship*, Buckingham: Open University Press.

Keith, L. and Morris, J. (1996) 'Easy targets: a disability rights perspective on the "children as carers" debate', in J. Morris (ed.), *Encounters with Strangers: Feminism and Disability*, London: The Women's Press, pp. 89–115.

Kempson, E. (1996) *Life on a Low Income*, York: York Publishing Services for the Joseph Rowntree Foundation.

Kidd Webster, S. (1988) *Service Delivery to Families in Wisconsin in which Parents have Mental Retardation*, Madison: Waisman Center on Mental Retardation and Human Development.

Kiernan, K. (1986) 'Transitions in young adulthood', in M. Murphy and J. Hobcraft (eds), *Population Research in Britain*, London: Population Investigation Committee.

Kohli, M. (1981) 'Biography: account, text and method', in D. Bertaux (ed.), *Biography and Society: The Life History Approach in the Social Sciences*, London: Sage Publications, pp. 61–75.

Korbin, J. (1987) 'Child maltreatment in cross-cultural perspective: vulnerable children and circumstances', in R. Gelles and J. Lancaster (eds), *Child Abuse and Neglect: Biosocial Dimensions*, New York: Aldine de Gruyter.

Kugel, R. and Parsons, M. H. (1967) *Changing the Course of Familial Retardation, DHEW Publication 440*, Washington DC: US Government Printing Office.

Labov, W. and Waletzky, J. (1967) 'Narrative analysis: oral versions of personal experience', in J. Helm (ed.), *Essays on the Verbal and Visual Arts*, San Francisco: American Ethnological Society.

Law Commission, The (1991) *Mentally Incapacitated Adults and Decision-Making: An Overview*, London: HMSO.

Lewis, O. (1961) *Children of Sanchez: Autobiography of a Mexican Family*, New York: Random House.

Lincoln, Y. and Denzin, N. (1994) 'The fifth moment', in N. Denzin and Y. Lincoln (eds), *Handbook of Qualitative Research*, Thousand Oaks, CA: Sage.

McFadyean, M. (1995) 'Why shouldn't this couple have a sex life?', *Marie Claire*, April, 52–58.

McGaw, S. (1993a) 'The Special Parenting Service – supporting parents with learning difficulties', *Disability, Pregnancy and Parenthood International*, 4, October, 8–10.

—— (1993b) 'Working with parents on parenting skills', in A. Craft (ed.), *Parents with Learning Disabilities*, Kidderminster: BILD.

McIntyre, K., White, D. and Yoast, R. (1990) *Resilience among High Risk Youth*, Wisconsin Clearinghouse: University of Wisconsin-Madison.

Magee, J. (1988) *A Professional's Guide to Older Adults' Life Review*, Lexington, MA: Lexington Books.

Maines, D. (1993) 'Narrative's moment and sociology's phenomena: toward a narrative sociology', *The Sociological Quarterly*, 34(1), 17–38.

Mandeville, H. (1992) 'Guiding principles for supporting families headed by parents with disabilities', in H. Mandeville (ed.), *Building the Foundation: Public Policy Issues in Supported Parenting. Supported Parenting Project*, Madison: Wisconsin Council on Developmental Disabilities.

Mercer, J. (1973) *Labeling the Mentally Retarded: Clinical and Social System Perspectives on Mental Retardation*, London: University of California Press.

Miller, W. (1994) 'State of Neglect: Part 3', *The Spokesman-Review*, Tuesday April 12, pp. H1–H4.

Morris, J. (1993) *Independent Lives? Community Care and Disabled People*, London: Macmillan.

Morrow, V. and Richards, M. (1996) *Transitions to Adulthood: A Family Matter?*, York: York Publishing Services for the Joseph Rowntree Foundation.

Mrazek, P. and Mrazek, D. (1987) 'Resilience in child maltreatment victims: a conceptual exploration', *Child Abuse and Neglect*, 11, 357–66.

National Children's Home (1992) *Deep in Debt: A Survey of Problems Faced by Low Income Families*, London: National Children's Home.

New York State Commission on Quality of Care for the Mentally Disabled (1993a) *Serving Parents who are Mentally Retarded: A Review of Eight Parenting Programs in New York State*, Albany, New York: New York State Commission on Quality of Care for the Mentally Disabled.

—— (1993b) *Parenting with Special Needs: Parents who are Mentally Retarded and their Children*, Albany, New York: New York State Commission on Quality of Care for the Mentally Disabled.

Oliver, J. (1977) 'Some studies of families in which children suffer maltreatment', in A. Franklin (ed.), *The Challenge of Child Abuse*, London: Academic Press.

Olsen, R. (1996) 'Young carers: challenging the facts and politics of research into children and caring', *Disability and Society*, 11(1), 41–54.

O'Neill, A. M. (1985) 'Normal and bright children of mentally retarded parents: the Huck Finn Syndrome', *Child Psychiatry and Human Development*, 15(4), 255–68.

Parker, G. and Olsen, R. (1995a) A plea to practitioners, *Community Care*, 14–20 September, 21.

—— (1995b) *A Sideways Glance at Young Carers*, University of Leicester: Nuffield Community Care Studies Unit.

Parker, T. (1991) *Life After Life*, London: Pan Books.

—— (1996) *Studs Terkel: A Life in Words*, London: Harper Collins.

Parton, N. (1991) *Governing the Family: Child Care, Child Protection and the State*, Basingstoke: Macmillan.

Peacock, J. and Holland, D. (1993) 'The narrated self: life stories in process', *Ethos*, 21(4), 367–83.

Petchesky, R. (1979) 'Reproduction, ethics and public policy: the federal regulations', *Hastings Center Report*, October, 29–41.

Plummer, K. (1983) *Documents of Life*, London: Allen and Unwin.

—— (1990) 'Herbert Blumer and the life history tradition', *Symbolic Interaction*, 13(2), 125–44.

Poulsen, M. (1993) 'Strategies for building resilience in infants and young children at risk', *Infants and Young Children*, 6(2), 29–40.

Prosser, J. (1992) *Child Abuse Investigations: The Families' Perspective*, Essex: Parents Against Injustice (PAIN).

Rapoport, R., Rapoport, R.N., Strelitz, Z. and Kew, S. (1977) *Fathers, Mothers and Others: Towards New Alliances*, London: Routledge and Kegan Paul.

Rickford, F. (1995) 'Beyond the call of duty', *Community Care*, 10–16 August, 20–1.

Rosenburg, S. and McTate, G. (1982) 'Intellectually handicapped mothers: problems and prospects', *Children Today*, Jan/Feb, 24–6, 37.

Rowland, G., Rowland, S. and Winter, R. (1990) 'Writing fiction as inquiry into professional practice', *Journal of Curriculum Studies*, 22(3), 291–3.

Runyan, W. (1984) *Life Histories and Psychobiography: Explorations in Theory and Method*, New York: Oxford University Press.

Rutter, M. (1974) 'Dimensions of parenthood: some myths and some suggestions', in Department of Health and Social Security (ed.), *The Family in Society: Dimensions of Parenthood*, London: HMSO.

—— (1987) 'Psychosocial resilience and protective mechanisms', *American Journal of Orthopsychiatry*, 57(3), 316–31.

Sandelowski, M. (1994) 'The proof is in the pottery: towards a poetic for qualitative inquiry', in J. Morse (ed.), *Critical Issues in Qualitative Research Methods*, London: Sage.

Scally, B. (1973) 'Marriage and mental handicap: some observations in Northern Ireland', in F. de la Cruz a. G. LaVeck (eds), *Human Sexuality and the Mentally Retarded*, New York: Brunner/Mazel.

Scheppele, K. (1989) 'Foreword: telling stories', *Michigan Law Review*, 87, 2073–98.

Schilling, R., Schinke, S., Blythe, B. and Barth, R. (1982) 'Child maltreatment and mentally retarded parents: is there a relationship?', *Mental Retardation*, 20(5), 201–9.

Schofield, G. (1996) 'Parental competence and the welfare of the child: issues for those who work with parents with learning difficulties and their children. A response to Booth and Booth', *Child and Family Social Work*, 1(2), 87–92.

Segal, J. and Simkins, J. (1993) *My Mum Needs Me*, Harmondsworth: Penguin.

Siegelman, C., Budd, E., Spenhel, C. and Schoenrock, C. (1981a) 'When in doubt, say yes: acquiescence in interviews with mentally retarded persons', *Mental Retardation*, April, 53–8.

Siegelman, C., Schoenrock, C., Winer, J., Spanhel, C., Hromas, S., Martin, P., Budd, E. and Bensberg, C. (1981b) 'Issues in interviewing mentally retarded persons: an empirical study', in C. Bruininks, B. Sigford and K. Lakin (eds), *Deinstitutionalization and Community Adjustment of Mentally Retarded People*, Monograph 4, Washington DC: American Association of Deficiency.

Siegelman, C., Budd, E., Winer, J., Schoenrock, C. and Martin, P. (1982) 'Evaluation alternative techniques of questioning mentally retarded persons', *American Journal of Mental Deficiency*, 86, 511–18.

Smith, C. and Pugh, G. (1996) *Learning to be a Parent: a Survey of Group-based Parenting Programmes*, London: Family Policy Studies Centre.

Snodgrass, P. (1992) 'How many? How much? Scarce resources and supported parenting', in H. Mandeville (ed.), *Building the Foundation: Public Policy Issues in Supported Parenting*, Madison: Wisconsin Council on Developmental Disabilities.

Sobsey, D. (1994) 'Sexual abuse in the lives of people with learning disabilities', *NAPSAC Bulletin No. 10*, December, 3–7.

Social Services Inspectorate (1995) *CI(95)12*, Vol. April, London: HMSO.

Spradley, J. (1979) *The Ethnographic Interview*, London: Holt, Rhinehart and Winston.

Stafford, D. (1992) *Children of Alcoholics: How a Parent's Drinking Can Affect Your Life*, London: Piatkus.

Steedman, C. (1990) *Childhood, Culture and Class in Britain*, London: Virago.

Stoneman, Z. (1989) 'Comparison groups in research on families with mentally retarded members: a methodological and conceptual review', *American Journal on Mental Retardation*, 94(3), 195–215.

Sweet, M. (1990) *Discovering the Parent's Language of Learning: An Educational Approach to Supporting Parents with Mental Retardation*, Madison: Wisconsin Council on Developmental Disabilities.

Thomas, W. and Znanieckis, F. (1927) *The Polish Peasant in Europe and America*, New York: Dover Publications.

Thompson, P. (1981) 'Life histories and the analysis of social change', in D. Bertaux (ed.), *Biography and Society*, London: Sage.

—— (1994) 'Tony Parker – writer and oral historian', *Oral History*, 25, Autumn, 64–73.

Thorpe, D. (1995) 'Some implications of recent child protection research', *Representing Children*, 8(3), 27–31.

Tithridge, E. (1995) 'A plea to policymakers', *Community Care*, 31 August–6 September, 15.

Tremblay, M. (1957) 'The key informant technique: a non-ethnographic application', *American Anthropologist*, 59, 688–98.

Tucker, M. and Johnson, O. (1989) 'Competence promoting versus competence inhibiting social support for mentally retarded mothers', *Human Organisation*, 48(2), 95–107.

Turk, V. and Brown, H. (1992) 'Sexual abuse and adults with learning disabilities', *Mental Handicap*, 20(2), 56–8.

—— (1993) 'Sexual abuse and adults with learning difficulties: results of a two-year incidence survey', *Mental Handicap*, 6(3), 193–216.

Turner, M. (1995) 'Voice of dissent', *Community Care*, 24–30 August, 14–15.

Tymchuk, A. (1990a) *Parents with Mental Retardation: A National Strategy*, SHARE/UCLA Parenting Project, Department of Psychiatry, School of Medicine, UCLA.

—— (1990b) 'Parents with mental retardation: a national strategy', *Journal of Disability Policy Studies*, 1(4), 44–56.

—— (1992) 'Predicting adequacy of parenting by people with mental retardation', *Child Abuse and Neglect*, 16(2), 165–78.

Tymchuk, A. and Feldman, M. (1991) 'Parents with mental retardation and their children: review of research relevant to professional practice', *Canadian Psychology*, 32(3), 486–96.

Ullmer, D., Kidd Webster, S. and McManus, M. (1991) *Cultivating Competence: Models of Support for Families Headed by Parents with Cognitive Limitations – A National Resource Directory*, Madison: Waisman Center on Mental Retardation and Human Development and Wisconsin Council on Developmental Disabilities.

Unger, O. and Howes, C. (1986) 'Mother-child interactions and symbolic play between toddlers and their adolescent or mentally retarded mothers', *The Occupational Therapy Journal of Research*, 8(4), 237–49.

Walker, R. (1981) 'On the uses of fiction in educational research – (and I don't mean Cyril Burt)', in D. Smetherham (ed.), *Practising Evaluation*, Driffield: Nafferton Books.

Warshaw, R. (1989) *I Never Called It Rape*, New York: Harper and Row.

Watt, N., David, J., Ladd, K. and Shamos, S. (1995) 'The life course of psychological resilience: a phenomenological perspective on deflecting life's slings and arrows', *The Journal of Primary Prevention*, 15(3), 209–46.

Webster, J. (1991) *Split in Two: Experiences of the Children of Schizophrenic Mothers*, Department of Social Work: University of Manchester.

Webster-Stratton, C. (1990) 'Stress: a potential disruptor of parents' perceptions and family interactions', *Journal of Clinical Child Psychology*, 19(4), 302–12.

Werner, E. (1989) 'High-risk children in young adulthood: A longitudinal study from birth to 32 years', *American Journal of Orthopsychiatry*, 59(1), 72–81.

—— (1993) 'Risk, resilience and recovery: perspectives from the Kauai Longitudinal Study', *Development and Psychopathology*, 5, 503–15.

Whitman, B. and Accardo, P. (eds) (1990) *When a Parent is Mentally Retarded*, Baltimore: Paul H. Brookes.

Whittemore, R., Langness, L. and Koegel, P. (1986) 'The life history approach to mental retardation', in L. Langness and H. Levine (eds), *Culture and Retardation*, Boston: Reidl Publishing Company.

Whyte, W. (1996) 'Qualitative sociology and deconstructionism', *Qualitative Inquiry*, 2(2), 220–9.

Williams, C. (1995) 'Clearer visions and equal value: achieving justice for victims with learning difficulties', in T. Philpot and L. Ward (eds), *Values and Visions: Changing Ideas in Services for People with Learning Difficulties*, London: Butterworth-Heinemann.

Williams, P. (1991) *The Alchemy of Race and Rights: The Diary of a Law Professor*, Cambridge: Harvard University Press.

Wolin, S. and Wolin, S. (1995) 'Resilience among youth growing up in substance-abusing families', *Pediatric Clinics of North America*, 42(2), 415–29.

Young, S., Young, B. and Ford, D. (1997) 'Parents with a learning disability: research issues and informed practice', *Disability and Society*, 12(1), 57–68.

Zetlin, A., Weisner T., and Gallimore, R. (1985) 'Diversity, shared functioning and the role of benefactors: a study of parenting by retarded persons', in S. Thurman (ed.), *Children of Handicapped Parents: Research and Clinical Perspectives*, New York: Academic Press.

Zimmerman, J. and Dickerson, V. (1994) 'Using a narrative metaphor: implications for theory and clinical practice', *Family Process*, 33(3), 233–45.